FITNESS TRAINING

Barry Davies BEM

 HarperCollins*Publishers*

HarperCollins Publishers

Westerhill Rd, Bishopbriggs Glasgow G64 2QT

www.**fire**and**water**.co.uk

First published 2001

Reprint 10 9 8 7 6 5 4 3 2 1 0

© Barry Davies 2001

ISBN 0 00 710229 1

Photo Credits: all photography © Barry Davies, except for images
on pp. 31, 34, 35, 50, 58, 72, 89 (top), 97, 122, 126, 132, 135, 208,
231, 232, © PhotoDisc 2001; on pp. 18, 23, 44, 46, 70, 76, 113,
124, 125, 134, 206, 222, © Artville 2001; and on pp. 6, 13, 81, 150,
158, 179, 180 © PS5 Ltd

Material in this book first appeared in the
Collins Gem *SAS Fitness*

Printed in Hong Kong by Midas

Contents

Programme Two

SAS Selection Techniques

Fitness Health and Injuries

Calorie-counted Menus and Food

Introduction

Without doubt the British Special Air Service (SAS) are the fittest military unit in the world. True, there may be specialist individuals in the USA or Russia who could compete and maybe win, but as a whole, the SAS come out tops. This is not just my opinion it is also that of most other special forces units around the world. How do they achieve this status? The answer is not pumping iron or working out in the gym for hours; it is a process called SAS Selection. Each volunteer who wishes to join must pass this course in order to be 'selected'.

I served with the SAS for 18 years, of which I am justly proud. During that time I took a keen interest in hillwalking and survival, subjects I continue to practice and write about. Likewise, when I'm not writing, I shoulder my rucksack and takes to the nearby mountains around my home in Spain. When back in Great Britain, I often visit the Brecon Beacons and surrounding Welsh mountains to walk the same routes which I covered when I attempted SAS Selection – though, it must be admitted, at a more sedate pace.

As far as possible this book describes a set of programmes based on the principles of diet and weight reduction and the fitness requirements of SAS Selection. The programmes have been adjusted from their strict military structure, thus allowing anyone from 16 to 60 to participate according to their individual capabilities. For those who simply want to lose weight the book will show them how, and for those who want to achieve a phenomenal degree of fitness there is a full schedule based around the SAS selection process.

The procedures start with techniques to evaluate your present physical condition, then lay out a simple but enjoyable routine starting with short strolls and eventually leading to marathon-type walks across beautiful countryside. Just like SAS Selection, which takes six months to accomplish, your routine will be a gradual process but one that will achieve long-term results. If you feel the need to regain fitness or to discover the benefits exercise brings, then this is the place to start. Your reward will be a longer life, more stamina, a feeling of wellbeing and a healthy body.

WHAT IS SAS SELECTION?

Any soldier who wishes to join the Special Air Service (SAS) must first pass an extremely tough process called 'Selection'. A series of endurance tests ensures that only the best candidates make it through to further training. To begin with, any soldier applying for

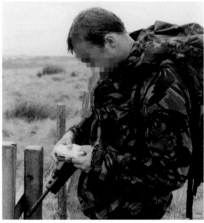

SAS selection requires that a soldier, who is already fit, pushes himself to the limit

Selection needs to have had at least three years service with a parent unit, so that at least the basics of military discipline and procedures are understood. Many people imagine that only soldiers can apply to be part of the SAS, however, the Selection is open to all men in all branches of the armed forces, as long as they have served for three years.

Every SAS candidate will have to earn his place by proving his abilities. In this way no-one is actually picked or chosen by anyone else – it is merely a process of survival of the fittest. This practice ensures that successful SAS candidates tend to be highly motivated, highly focused individuals who are still able to work as part of a team. Once Selection has been passed, the candidate must then give up any rank previously held in his parent regiment and will once more become a trooper.

The Selection process itself takes place, for the main part, in the Brecon Beacons in South Wales. The Beacons are not particularly high, but the constant weather changes mean that they can be dangerous. More than one soldier has met his death through hypothermia. A prospective candidate needs to put himself through some sort of training schedule to get fit a long time before he gets to Hereford. The best way of building endurance is to go on increasingly long walks with a medium-sized rucksack. However, a good knowledge of map reading is also essential as the candidate will be required to navigate his own routes across the test sections.

The first obstacle encountered by the candidate is 'Test Week', which comes at the end of the first phase of SAS Selection. It is a week designed to test individual stamina and fitness and its gruelling nature often means that several candidates drop out every day. From my own experience, one of the best ways to make it through this week, apart from being fit, is to eat as much food as possible, especially breakfast. The finale of the week is a killer of an exercise known as the 'endurance march'. For this, the remaining candidates are expected to cover 25 miles (40km) in 20 hours carrying a rifle and a 55-lb (25-kilo) bergen, and, of course, the route is anything but flat.

Summer Selection means that the candidate will be at risk of severe dehydration, while Winter Selection carries the threat of hypothermia. The soldier is expected to be aware of these dangers and to adequately safeguard against them. But whatever the time of year, he will still need to carry adequate protection against any sudden changes in weather. Once the candidate reaches the end of the course within the allotted time, he will find army trucks waiting to take him back to base. The worst of the physical tests may be over, but there will still be much more training to come over the next few months before he will be able to call himself an SAS soldier.

Don't worry, no-one is going to make you do SAS Selection, but we are going to incorporate many of its principles into our own fitness programme. These principles involve weight loss, fitness and endurance, all achieved through healthy eating, drinking and aerobic exercise. Whereas the SAS start off with professional soldiers, many readers of this book will need to find their own fitness level first.

Fitness Training has four main levels. First, it concentrates on those people who are very overweight and are unable to exercise properly; those that consider themselves to be in this category will need to start with the Weight-loss Programme (see p. 57). The other three levels are based on simple fitness exercise programmes. The first concentrates on general health and fitness, while the other two are designed around the Special Forces Briefing Course and SAS Selection. Although these are modified for civilian use the routes are extremely gruelling. It is up to the individual to decide at which point they will enter a particular fitness programme, but I highly recommend that everyone undergo the health and fitness test prior to any strenuous exercise.

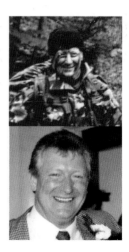

Before I became a writer in my late 40s, I was extremely fit, running at least 20 miles a week and walking most weekends. However, along with the opportunity to change lifestyles, came the endless hours sitting in front of a computer (around 12 hours a day). Now some six years down the line and despite sticking to a rigid diet my weight has shot up to some 16 stone 7lbs (104 kg), simply due to lack of exercise. So during the three months it takes to write this book I have decided to participate in my own fitness programme to achieve a better weight and standard of fitness. My progress is accurately recorded throughout this book and stands as testimony to its viability. I will apply the same motivation and persistence to exercise as I do to my writing. (Before and after photographs along with a periodic weight check will be my affidavit to such.)

WARNING

➤ The aim of this book is to help create a diet and fitness plan appropriate to an individual's current health and fitness levels. Everyone can aim for the same standards, with age, time and motivation being the only differences. This book is tailored to those of normal eating habits and does not cater for people on a restricted or specialized diet. It is not suitable for vegetarians or vegans. The diets and exercises described are for use in circumstances where safety or health are not put at risk. The author and the publishers will not accept any responsibility or legal liability for any health and fitness recommendations or diets used in this book. Individuals with heart and cardiovascular conditions, diabetes hypoglycaemia, kidney disease, stroke, gout, the very elderly, growing children, adolescents, pregnant women or anyone under medical care for any other condition must follow the dietary (including daily calorific intake) recommendations given to them or approved by their doctor, dietician, nutritionist or other qualified health professional.

A Fit and Healthy Body

DEFINING OUR AIM

It is sad to say that less than 30 per cent of the European population exercise on a regular basis; in the USA the figure is even lower. In itself this would not be so bad, but when you add a poor diet, the body becomes unfit and unhealthy. This is somewhat surprising given the benefits of a fit and healthy body. Improved cardiovascular fitness helps fight against heart disease, and weight loss improves energy levels as well as providing a feeling of wellbeing and a longer life expectancy.

How is this done? To start with you must ask yourself: 'What do I want to achieve?' Do you want to be slimmer? If so, by how much? Do you want to be fitter, and for what reason, e.g. to simply gain more energy or to run a marathon? Then ask yourself: 'What must I do to achieve that aim?' You must all answer these questions honestly.

The next requirement is to set yourself a realistic target, and a time span over which you can sensibly accomplish that target. In doing this consider how long it took you to gain weight or become unfit. Even with the best will in the world it's going to take a long time to reach your desired goal. Think about your age; we are all getting older and thus slowing down. Do you have the motivation? There can be no progress without a commitment to a long-term diet and exercise routine; many start off at a cracking pace but give up after a few days. There must be a determination to diet and exercise, in the same way as you commit yourself to go to work each day. Make time for your exercise programme and build it into your daily routine. This is particularly important during the first four weeks.

GETTING STARTED

Some basic knowledge of how the human body works is helpful if we are to get fit. We need to understand the benefits of proper nutrition and just how food affects the whole body. In particular it is crucial to know how the blood takes oxygen and nutrients via the heart to our muscles. These cause the muscles to develop healthily and to be able to stretch and contract properly, which, of course, enables us to move. In order for our body to be at its most efficient and vitalized, these processes must also be able to work at their optimum capacity.

However, it must also be understood that there are some differences in the physiological make-up of men and women, which must be detailed before we start.

DIFFERENCES BETWEEN THE SEXES

This book is aimed at both men and women and as

such, the diet and exercise programmes are meant for both sexes. But there are differences which need to be taken into account when planning fitness goals.

Body Mass

As a rule, most men have a greater body mass than women. For example, an average 18-year-old male will have a height of about 5 feet 8 inches (1.72 m) and will weigh around $10^1/_2$ stone (66.15 kg). An average 18-year-old woman, on the other hand, will have a height of about 5 feet 5 inches and a weight of around 9 stone (57 kg). This difference will affect the amount of muscular strength between men and women.

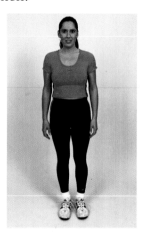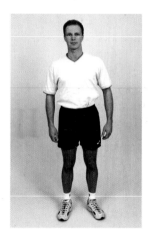

Muscles and Bones

In general, men have approximately 50 per cent more muscle mass than women as well as a greater bone mass. This means that although women are not as strong they do have greater flexibility.

Fat

The female body accumulates a greater amount of body fat than the male body. It is usually distributed in the buttocks, arms and thighs, whereas in men it tends to be on the back, chest and stomach.

Heart Size and Rate

The heart of the average man is 25 per cent larger than that of the average woman and so is able to pump out more blood with every beat. This also means that men have a lower resting heart rate (five to eight beats a minute slower) than women.

Lung Capacity

As with the heart, the lung capacity in men is about 25–30 per cent greater than that in women. This enables men to take in more oxygen when exercising.

THE HUMAN BODY

Our size and shape are mainly determined by our skeleton, which is genetically inherited and sustained by normal growth. While there is little we can do about our skeletal frame, fat and muscle can be altered because they respond to exercise. The composition of the average human body is as follows, though the percentages vary with age and gender:

➤ bone and minerals: 6–8%
➤ muscle and other lean tissue: 10–20%
➤ body fat: 15–25%
➤ water: 55–60%

The Skeleton

Our skeleton is what provides the framework for the rest of our body, both supporting and protecting various parts of it. The size and shape of our skeleton is genetically inherited but it can be influenced by nutrition and disease. It contains a total of 206 bones, half of which are concentrated in the intricate structures of the hands and feet. Various types of joints connect one bone to another, making the body

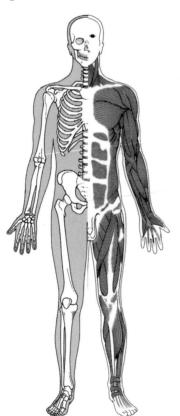

flexible and able to perform a wide range of movements. Male and female skeletons are similar but with a few slight differences: the bones of the male are heavier and thicker; while women have a shallower and wider pelvis As already mentioned, the skeleton cannot be altered (unless through disease, injury or surgery), but we can affect fat and muscle through diet and exercise.

Muscle

There are about 650 muscles in the body, generally attached to the skeleton by tendons. They make up over 20–25 per cent of the total body weight Exercise develops muscles and muscle groups either for stamina or for strength, depending on what kind of exercise is employed and therefore dictates our outer body shape.

Body fat

Body fat stores unused energy and is essential to a healthy body, but if it becomes excessive it can be unsightly and unhealthy. Women naturally carry more body fat than men, but both increase their body fat percentage with age. As a rough guide see below.

AVERAGE BODY FAT

Age	17–20	21–27	28–39	40+
Male	20%	23%	26%	28%
Female	28%	30%	32%	34%

Body Water

Water is the largest single component of the human body; the blood itself is 80 per cent water. The body has no way of storing water and so it constantly needs to be replaced by drinking fluids. This is why water is so important to health, and without it death will occur in about three days. Normal water loss occurs through the natural processes of respiration, urination and perspiration. Ideally, fluid intake should be equal to fluid loss; when we perspire or urinate we should drink in order to replace that loss on a regular basis.

The Heart

Of all the muscles in the body, the heart is the most important, for without it we would die. While we are alive, it works ceaselessly, pumping blood around the body; oxygen and nutrients are delivered to vital organs, bones and muscle, and waste products are carried away. The heart muscle is extremely efficient. It has four chambers: two of these deal with pumping de-oxygenated blood to the lungs for re-oxygenation; while the other two receive the blood back from the lungs and pump it around the body. During activity or exercise, the heart needs to work harder to enable it to pump out more blood to the muscles. If these muscles do not receive the oxygen they require, they soon tire and build up waste products, such as lactic acid. Therefore, for improved fitness, the heart rate needs to be raised to 80 per cent of its maximum capability.

Like the rest of the body, the heart is vulnerable to injury and disease and the effects of these are potentially life-threatening. Heart, or cardiovascular disease can come in many forms and may be either mild or serious. Some forms are congenital but most are brought on by an unhealthy lifestyle and occur later on in life. A heart attack can be caused by diseased coronary arteries, cardiomyopathy, hypertension and valvular heart disease. Such conditions may be avoided by sensible diet and exercise. The twentieth century has seen many advances in the area of heart medicine, whether it be new drugs, pacemakers or surgical procedures. Many sufferers of heart disease have had their symptoms relieved or even eliminated altogether. However, the best cure is still prevention and the only way to do that is to keep fit.

The two main factors affecting the heart are diet and exercise. A poor diet over a long period causes a substance called atheroma to build up in the arteries. Eventually this wax-like substance will block the arteries and so interrupt the blood supply to that part of

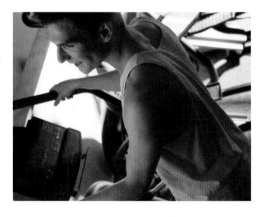

the body. A blockage in the coronary arteries can cause chest cramps (angina) or even a heart attack. As with any muscle the heart will respond and improve with exercise. A normal pulse rate is around

65–70 beats per minute. The resting pulse, taken when we first wake up, is normally a little lower. This resting pulse rate falls the fitter we become. In real terms this means the heart rate of an unfit person doing exercise will be around 120 beats per minute. In a fit person doing the same exercise it will be greatly reduced to around 85–90 beats per minute. In the course of a minute's activity the hearts of both the fit and unfit person will pump the same volume of blood, the difference being that the fit person's heart will need less beats to do it.

The unfit heart will simply beat faster to compensate for the exercise while the fit heart meets the demand by increasing the stroke volume – thus the fit heart does a lot less work. Getting fit also improves the blood flow around the body by lessening the resistance in the vessels and therefore lowering the blood pressure. A combination of high blood pressure and poor diet is the main cause of heart attacks.

The Respiratory System

The respiratory system takes in oxygen from the air outside and supplies it to the blood. It is also responsible for the expulsion of waste gases such as carbon monoxide, which are a by-product of the respiratory process. Air is taken in through the nose and down to the lungs via the windpipe, or trachea. At the top of the trachea is located the voicebox, or larynx. Further down in the chest, the trachea branches into two tubes, called bronchi which lead into the left and right lungs. Within the lungs, the bronchi divide into smaller and smaller tubes called bronchioles. These all carry the air to tiny little chambers at the end of the bronchioles, called alveoli. It is in these chambers that the oxygen in the air is able to pass through the thin membranes of the walls and into the blood capillaries beyond. Here the oxygen molecules attach themselves to blood cells which then become re-oxygenated. In the same way, waste gases are able to cross from the blood and into the alveoli to be eventually expelled on the next outbreath. The lungs are able to inhale and exhale air due to the contraction and expansion of the thoracic cavity. This contraction and expansion is due for the most part to the workings of a large, thin sheet of muscle located just below the ribcage – the diaphragm, as well as the intercostal and abdominal muscles. The ribs themselves act to support and protect the thoracic cavity.

LEARNING TO BREATHE

If you have not exercised for a long time or are very overweight, you will have trouble breathing. Your lungs will need to expand again, which takes time and if you begin too quickly, you will suffer laboured breathing and chest pain. Control your breathing as follows:

➤ exhale fully, then inhale slowly to the count of 10;

➤ exhale to the same count;

➤ repeat this three times – it has an amazing effect.

Once the burning pain has receded, carry on with the exercise but at a much reduced level of effort. If you still have chest pain remains, cease the activity and consult your doctor.

Fresh air feeds the blood that in turn feeds the muscle and brain. Work out in an area where the air is clean and vary the exercises so that the lungs operate at a variety of speeds. Once you have achieved a standard of breathing where you feel no undue pain or stress in the chest cavity, try to improve slightly by pushing yourself in short but vigorous exercise. The amount and quality of air we breathe has a direct effect on our health, as with the water we consume, purity and volume make for a healthy body.

A CHANGE IN LIFESTYLE

There are other factors we must take into consideration when assessing our fitness which are not always readily apparent but are just as important. The major factor is our lifestyle. Work is the dominant part of almost everyone's lifestyle, with other periods such as sleep and leisure time falling into step. All of which make up our daily routine. Changes to our lifestyles, our routines, can be difficult and often stressful, for example, a change of job. It is hard to uproot yourself and to head off in a new direction, and getting fit will certainly involve a great deal of alteration to your daily habits. However, concentrating on the benefits of being fit should provide you with the necessary motivation and determination to break your bad habits, and make getting fit and staying fit a central part of your way of life.

Bad Habits

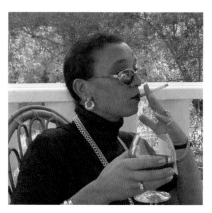

Bad habits can be hard to break but the benefits will make it worth it in the end.

We all have some bad habits, such as excessive eating, drinking, smoking, or even, in some cases, drug abuse and dependency. No matter how you argue the case for alcohol or soft drugs, neither one of these promote a healthy body or satisfactory lifestyle. What we must recognize in ourselves is that the habit is there. If, like many people, you suffer from two or more habits then you have real problems. For example, if you drink and smoke excessively, the odds are you will die well before your time. The odd drink doesn't do much harm, but a build-up of alcohol in the system over years will cause irreversible damage to the liver, eventually leading to death. Excess alcohol also has a deleterious effect on the heart, kidneys, brain and other organs. There is no doubt about it that alcohol in large amounts is a poison to the system. Another toxic habit is smoking. The tar contained in cigarettes is drawn into the lungs and will eventually cause many major health problems. Heart disease, lung cancer, throat and mouth cancer, and thrombosis are all associated with smoking and all have a high death rate. Neither do you need to be a smoker to end up with the same disorders: recent research has shown that those people who constantly breathe in other people's smoke are also at risk.

If you feel that you could have a problem, do something about it. Plan to make a fresh start but do it slowly and tackle one problem at a time, whether it is your diet, smoking, drinking, stress or lack of exercise, and set yourself a simple goal to start with.

The Benefits of Fitness

Health and fitness help promote a long active life and, providing no major accident befalls you, if you resolve to make diet and exercise a long-term option then there is no reason why you should not achieve that aim. Fitness must become a part of your life, and the younger you start the better your body reacts. Fitness not only controls your weight, but there is good evidence that you will be less prone to many life-threatening diseases, such as heart disease. Getting fit helps you to enjoy life a lot more; you feel better, have more energy and look a whole lot better too. The good thing about exercise is that you start to feel the benefits from day one. After four weeks you will find you have more energy and you will sleep better. Three months down the line and you will have

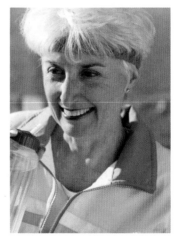

improved your personal appearance, you will feel good and should have a lot fewer health problems. A year later, providing you are still keeping to your programme, your whole life will have changed and you will feel a different person.

Motivation

Motivation is the process through which people provoke, endure and control what happens in their lives. In this case we are provoked to become fitter. For many of us this means having to endure a strict regime of diet and exercise while controlling the rest of our lives. One thing I promise you, no matter at what point in life you start your fitness programme, if you endure, you will reap the benefits. First you must understand why you want to be fit. For example:

➤ Do you consider yourself obese?
➤ Are you in poor health or do you have shortage of breath?
➤ Are you afraid that your partner is losing interest?
➤ Do you wish to feel attractive to others?
➤ Do you have the desire to run a marathon?

Study other people of the same age that you admire. What qualities do they have that you do not? Whatever it is, in the end it comes down to confidence and motivation and if they can do it, so can you. So how do you become motivated? In this case simply make yourself a promise: 'I will get fit.' True, that's the easy bit. Next you need the confidence to endure. Determination will help you on track – remember why you started this fitness programme in the first place.

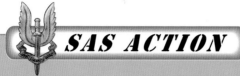

SAS ACTION

➤ SAS selection is hard; there is no other way to say it. The basis of the selection system is there to ensure that the valuable training time is only spent on the very best recruits. In the dictionary, the verb "select" means to pick out the best or most suitable. The adjective means chosen for excellence. At Hereford nobody picks or chooses the candidate, they must earn their place. It's more a case of the individual selecting himself. It's what makes the SAS unique: a group of individuals with the capacity to act as one.

Determination

For most of us getting fit is a long-term project, and your determination will require a boost from time to time. You may feel that all this training is getting you nowhere; why should you bother to continue? To this I can offer only one answer: get the first month over with, then your daily training will become second nature and before long you will start to enjoy it.

Coping with stress

Stress is an emotional and physical response to situations and events which we find unpleasant, worrying, annoying, frightening and so on; from traffic snarl ups to the death of a loved one, from a visit to the dentist to losing a job. However, it is an essential and natural part of life.

In many instances our body's reaction to it can be beneficial. Muscles become tense, increasing their flexibility and the breathing rate increases, so supplying more oxygen to the muscles. Sugars are discharged into the bloodstream to provide energy, and the heart rate increases to supply more blood to the muscles. Beads of sweat will break out from the skin, in readiness to cool the body as it overheats from strained exertion. If the stress is temporary, these symptoms will soon subside. However, if you remain in a 'wound-up' state over a long period, the biochemical state of your body will change and become unbalanced. It is thought that constant stress is the cause or at least a contributing factor in a range of health problems, such as temporary mental illness, certains cancers and heart disease. Fitness is one of the best ways of combating its effects.

Age

No matter how strong your determination, motivation and confidence, the body ages and there is a point at which stage the ageing process will simply deny any further progress. As we get older we lose muscle weight, flexibility and the bones become brittle.

When this will occur will differ in everyone, but it is often related to an individual's lifestyle. For some it will come early, while for others it may be in their seventies or eighties. There is little we can do about our age, but there is a lot we can do about showing it. To act young is to be young. Age brings many changes to our body but to some degree exercise and a healthy diet can counter the worst of these. Many men and women in their seventies and eighties still run marathons.

We normally reach the peak of fitness at around 30, and from there on in it's a steady decline. This decline is slow to start with, only making a difference in physical fitness around the age of 40. This is a time when the demands of work and family life are at there height. There are many reasons for this: stress, mostly money related, teenage children and divorce are but a few.

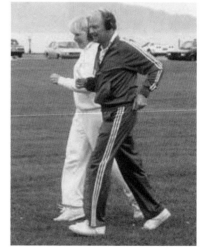

Medically, the older we get the less blood the heart is able to pump per beat, which lowers physical ability and performance. Additionally, body fat increases while muscle mass decreases. The result being a drop in cardio-respiratory efficiency as well as muscle strength and endurance. Flexibility also suffers. Regular workouts can change this to the point where a 60-year-old man can achieve the same cardio-respiratory fitness as an inactive 30-year-old.

How physical training affects you will depend on your age and length of inactivity. If you have been a keen and regular exerciser, then you should simple continue with your own routine. However, if you have been inactive for a long time, you will need to take things very easy. That's not to say its impossible for an older person to get fit, it just takes longer.

Understanding Weight Control

In order to achieve fitness we must also understand the effect of food in relation to our weight. This is equally as important as exercise, because if an individual is vastly overweight they cannot exercise sufficiently enough to make any significant difference to their fitness. Eating appropriately is critical for the proper growth and functioning of our bodies. Understanding why we eat and the properties of what we eat is, in the long term, more important than exercise, but the best option is a balanced combination of both.

DIET AND EXERCISE

By reducing your calorific intake (eating less) and increasing calorie burn by expending more energy (exercising), you should realistically expect a weight loss in the region of one or two pounds a week. It is not wise to try and lose weight by dieting alone, however, because the body will begin to think it is being starved and will compensate in other ways. It does this by slowing down its metabolic rate and as a result tends to conserve fat so that weight is lost very slowly. It is also a myth that diets should be a form of starvation. The body needs a minimum of around

1500 calories a day to function properly, though certain people may require more or less due to special circumstances. Also, it is nutritionally sensible that the calories should be spread out over all the major food groups.

Crash diets involving food regimes that work on a smaller calorie intake a day are best avoided as these tend not to produce lasting weight loss. They simply deplete body water and lean muscle tissue rather than body fat. The best diets take time and are usually combined with some form of exercise so that muscle tissue is maintained while fat is reduced. Aerobic exercise is the best type of exercise for reducing fat as the oxygen used is also necessary for the metabolization of fat into energy. Exercises considered to be aerobic are: jogging; swimming; walking; dancing; aerobics; cycling; stair-climbing; cross-country skiing; rowing; and skipping. Whichever diet-and-exercise method you intend to use, it should be carried out in a safe and sensible fashion.

WHAT IS FOOD?

In order that we can live, the body must have air, water and food. As a guide, without air we will begin to die within four minutes, without water within four days and without food forty days. Air and breathing have already been covered in the previous chapter, and so now we will look at how food and water affect the body.

The food that fuels the body falls into four main groups:

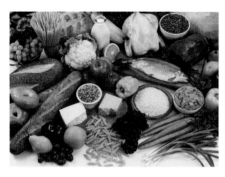

➤ Fruit and vegetables

➤ Cereals and breads

➤ Dairy products

➤ Meats

The four food groups

EATING HABITS AND CRAVINGS

We eat when our bodies crave food either through hunger orbecause there is a chemical deficiency in our energy balance. We also eat for the pleasure of it, for the taste or socially, or we eat because we are feeling stressed. In the first instance, once our body is used to eating at regular intervals, such as breakfast, lunch and dinner, signals are sent to the brain close to those times demanding replenishment, and we interpret these signals as a craving. If we go without food for a long period of time, the signals become more intense until the craving is satisfied. It is known that a fall in blood sugar levels triggers the signal to eat, although a deficiency in one particular chemical, such as salt, will also cause a demand for replenishment. Failure to obey the warning may result in symptoms such as dizziness and weakness.

On average Westerners eat about a tonne of food each year, and usually it is a constant intake of high-energy and fatty food – and therein lies the problem. Eating a lot of food will not make you fat overnight; it

takes time, years in many cases, for the fat to build.
Equally, eating very little will not make you thin in a
matter of days and your body weight will not fall
dramatically. That is why when people start a diet
their weight varies very little and they may become
disheartened. The secret to maintaining a stable body
weight is to eat uniformly, matching your energy loss
to your energy intake.

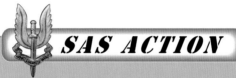

SAS ACTION

➤ At the age of twenty-two, SAS selection
  robbed my body of every ounce of surplus
  fat. Many of the candidates would skip
  breakfast for the sake of an extra half
  hour in bed. During the day the long
  marches caused physical exhaustion to
  the point where the body begins to
  reject food by making you vomit. Eating
  a good calorie-packed breakfast was my
  way of making it through the day.

GUIDELINES FOR HEALTHY EATING

You should try to eat a wide variety of different foods
from each main food group (see p. 33), with lots of
fruit and vegetables but smaller amounts of meats and
other fatty foods. A wider variety of foods satisfies the
appetite quicker and reduces the need for bulk. This

variety will help provide the body with a sufficient amount of fats, proteins, carbohydrates, vitamins, minerals and water. While all are beneficial to health, the fat content of food is the most significant. The value of the food we consume is defined by its calorific value. Foods differ in the calorific energy they provide depending on the amount of fats, protein and so on that they contain.

Once the principles of good nutrition are under-stood, maintaining a healthy, balanced diet becomes easy. If the guidelines are kept to and food is selected sensibly, it will provide the body with all the nutrients it requires to stay healthy and without gaining weight. Ideally, we should eat three meals a day, perhaps with a healthy snack, such as fruit, in between. If such a regime is followed, most adults would not need any vitamin or mineral supplements, however few of us stick to such a regime therefore additional vitamins and mineral become essential to well being.

Eating for your age

Where possible we should eat foods that best satisfy the body's requirements, but remember that these requirements change with age. For example, a teenager who goes to an all-night rave is going to need a different food intake to that, say, of an office worker in his forties who spends most of his free time surfing the internet (and a lot do).

Teenager

You can never start good eating habits early enough.

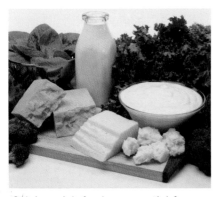

Calcium-rich foods – essential for gowing teenagers

Unfortunately, although many experts disapprove of a diet based entirely on fast food, which is undoubtedly the preferred choice of the average teenager, not enough is done to educate or provide an alternative. Teenagers are still growing, therefore their calcium intake is very important and low-fat diary products best fill this requirement, but it should be stressed that dairy food high in saturated fats should be avoided. Iron is also important in growing teenagers, particularly girls because they excrete as much as 2 mg per day during their periods. The best source of iron is blood, but getting a teenage girl to eat black-pudding or liver would be an uphill struggle, and so more acceptable alternatives are shell food, cereal or vegetables.

Adults 20 to 40

This can be the most problematic period because we start to gain weight, take less exercise and become less active, while stress and responsibilities increase. It is a good idea to replace as much red meat with white meat or fish. Increase the amount of cereal, wholemeal bread and vegetables in your diet. Use olive oil instead of butter or margarine for dressings and cooking. While olive oil is heavy in calories they are the right kind of calories and will help reduce the possibility of colon cancer. Control your eating habits; have a good break-fast, medium lunch and small dinner. Take multivitamin tablets as these help strengthen bones and maintain overall health.

Adults 40 to 65

A healthy diet at this stage is vital to sustaining the immune system. A poor diet increases the risk of coronary heart disease and cancer. Oestrogen levels also begin to drop, leaving the heart susceptible to disease. You should increase the amount of antioxidants in your diet, such as selenium and vitamins E and C, or increase the amount of gar-

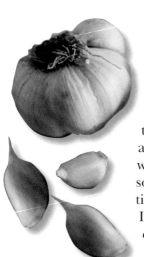

lic in your food. Another, perhaps more attractive, way is to drink a couple of glasses of red wine every day, although reducing the amount of hard alcohol consumed will also prove beneficial. Equally beneficial would be to try and eat your food without any salt, after about a week you will not miss it and the reduced sodium will prevent water retention and high blood pressure. Increase the amount of fruit you eat – the body thrives on simple unmodified foods such as apples oranges and bananas.

What We Eat

The range and general quality of food has improved dramatically over the past 30 years, but this improvement has also increased the amount of appetizing, high-energy foods available and the desire to consume more. This can be clearly seen in the growth of supermarkets and the huge variety of food products they sell. In the 1950s our mothers would go to the grocers and choose from a comparatively limited selection of food, today we simply push our trolley down the aisle past a seemingly never-ending display of mouth-watering products. Today, it is not just a matter of buying something to eat but increasingly it's a case of 'oh that looks nice lets try it'.

To maintain a well-balanced diet there are a few guidelines to follow when shopping for food:

FOOD BUYING GUIDELINES

➤   Buy fresh food whenever possible, frozen if not.

➤   Select foods which can be grilled or boiled (avoid fried food).

➤   Avoid chocolate, ice cream and anything with a high sugar or salt content.

➤   Skip the aisle with the high-calorie soft drinks and spirits.

➤ Limit the amount of pre-cut chips.

➤ Avoid high-calorie 'pick-at' foods, such as peanuts.

➤ Make a shopping list and stick to it.

➤ Increase the amount of vegetables you eat and decrease the meats.

➤ Buy more fruit.

➤ Buy spring water and plenty of it.

Food Usage

The bulk of what we eat falls into proteins, fats and carbohydrates, which make up over half of our daily energy requirement. The energy requirement is measured in calories. For a woman the average intake should be 2000 calories a day, for a man 2500. The ideal combination is 15 per cent protein, 35 per cent fat and 50 per cent carbohydrates. This roughly equates to:

➤ Breakfast: cereal with banana and skimmed milk, cup of tea/coffee with one sugar.

➤ Lunch: tuna sandwich, can of coke, piece of fruit.

➤ Dinner: lean steak, vegetables, cheese and biscuits.

➤ Drink: two measures of alcohol.

The importance of eating a well-balanced diet both in terms of differing foods and total quantity must be fully understood, especially when it comes to fat.

Fats

Fats are made up of carbon and hydrogen molecules. They differ in composition, but when considering health they fall into two main categories: saturated and unsaturated. In either case the more fat a food contains the higher the calorific value. The difference is that saturated fat will increase the cholesterol level in the blood, whereas unsaturated fats will help reduce it. The densest saturation takes place when a carbon atom is encompassed by the utmost number of hydrogen atoms possible. In general animal fats are highly saturated, while vegetable oil contains unsaturated fats. For example, butter is around 80 per cent fat of which 50–60 per cent is saturated, while a margarine high in polyunsaturates is 100 per cent fat of which only 25 per cent is saturated. It should be noted that we need to consume all fats, albeit in the correct amount, if we wish to maintain a healthy body.

Excessive Fat Intake

If we, as many of us do, eat until we have had our fill and ignore the content of the food we consume, then we will certainly include an excessive amount of fat in our diet. Excess fat makes your heart and vital organs work a lot harder. It blocks the arteries and restricts the blood flow, is unsightly and extremely heavy.

Body fat is accumulated over a number of years.

There is a slow build up of layer upon layer until we cannot ignore the problem. Even at this stage few people do anything about it other than to buy clothes in larger sizes.

An increase in the amount of fat slows the body's functions, making the problem self-perpetuating as physical exercise becomes difficult, unappealing and even dangerous. Carrying surplus fat around also has a marked influence on breathing, which becomes ragged, short and rasping, preventing the body's metabolization of fat-burning oxygen.

Cholesterol

Cholesterol is a waxy substance that is vital to the walls of all body cells. Most cholesterol is manufactured by the body, mostly in the liver, with less than 15 per cent coming from our dietary intake. The more fat we eat, the more the liver is encouraged to produce cholesterol. Cholesterol has two forms: higher density lipoprotein (HDL) – 'good cholesterol'; and lower density lipoprotein (LDL) – 'bad cholesterol', the difference being the amount of fat-laden protein attached. These are distributed around the body via the bloodstream and the related amounts of HDL and LDL are a good indicator of likely heart disease. It has been found that an increased amount of HDL has a beneficial effect on the body. To some degree this can be achieved by reducing the amount of saturated fats we consume in our diet. Additionally, HDL can be increased through exercise, though you will need to walk a total of at least 25 miles a week to produce a higher HDL level.

Protein

Proteins form the structure of our bodies and without them we would dissolve into one big heap of goo. All our cells are protein-based; they are essential for growth, cell repair and tissue replacement. Proteins are constructed from amino acids, so to make new proteins we need to eat foods that contain amino acids, such as fish, meat and eggs.

Carbohydrate

Carbohydrates contain atoms of carbon, hydrogen and oxygen in different configurations. These produce sugars and starches, the elements necessary for producing energy for movement in the body. When a carbohydrate is digested it breaks down into simple sugars, such as glucose, which can then be used by the body as fuel to provide energy for all the metabolic processes. Glucose does not just go straight into the blood; some of it goes to the liver where it is converted to glycogen and stored for future energy needs. Once these stores are depleted, the body will draw upon its fat and protein reserves to provide it with the fuel it needs. Carbohydrates also contain an amount of dietary fibre, but this is mostly removed during the body's processing of the food. Examples of foods high in carbohydrates are potatoes, wholemeal bread, pasta, rice and fruit.

CALORIE INTAKE

We eat food to sustain our bodily processes, which account for a little over two-thirds of what we consume, the remainder being used to fuel external activity, such as walking, working and exercise. If we do not eat enough while exercising extensively, we will burn off body fat – our body fuel reserves. If we eat too much and do not exercise then our fat reserves will get larger. Make sure that your daily calorie intake is matched to your needs; you will need more food if you intend to go hillwalking than if you are sitting at a desk all day. The secret of maintaining a sensible weight is all down to balancing energy needs. The exact amount of food, and therefore calories, required to maintain an even balance will depend on our age and lifestyle. The older we become, the less energy is required to maintain body muscle. As our lifestyle changes, due to work practices and social activities, so will the amount of calories required to maintain that balance.

AUTHOR'S NOTE

➤ Many people talk about the benefits of the Mediterranean Diet and until I moved to Spain recently, I thought this was just one more 'fix the fat' type diets. However I was wrong: the Spanish really do live longer, and not only that, they remain fitter and more agile in their old age. The reason has to be their environment and their food. Among the main exports of Spain's Mediterranean

(contd)

AUTHOR'S NOTE

coastline are fish, red wine, oranges and olive related products. The country also offers some of the purest air and water in the worl, added to which the sun shines almost every day.

➤ This healthy phenomenon stems from the people living on what they produce, and thus eating a healthy diet. For example, they eat mainly fish and white meat, lots of salad, use olive oil for dressings and cooking; this is often washed down with red wine, fruit juice or spring water. In essence, the near perfect diet on a daily basis.

CALORIE BURN

A calorie is one-thousandth part of the heat needed to heat one litre of water by one degree centigrade. It is the energy value by which foods are measured when consumed. For fitness terms a calorie is the measured amount of energy that is released as heat when food is metabolized by the body. The amount of calories in various foods and drinks vary, but as a rough guide:

➤ Fat contains nine calories per gram.

➤ Alcohol seven calories per gram.

➤ Carbohydrates and protein four calories per gram.

The amount of energy an individual burns during a

single day will depend on their activity and to some degree their exercising body weight. Most of us follow a daily routine which comprises of work, rest and play. For example, we all sleep for roughly 8 hours during which time the calorie burn is around 65 cph (calories per hour). As our work practices differ so will our calorie burn. For example, an office worker's will differ from that, say, of a farm worker. Most of us also spend a couple of hours travelling either to and from work, to the shops or to some leisure activity. The rest of our time is taken up with relaxation and personal activity.

Our personal activity time is where we can make a major difference to our daily calorie burn. For example, a sluggish teacher who spends his activity time 'surfing the net' in the evening will have a total calorie burn of around 2760 calories per day, while a waitress who enjoys dancing will average over 4000 calories per day.

TYPICAL DAILY CALORIE BURN

➤ **Sleeping:**

  65 cph x 8 hours = 520 calories

➤ **Desk work, driving:**

  100 cph x 8 hours = 800 calories

➤ **Hospital worker, school teacher:**

  200 cph x 8 hours = 1600 calories

➤ **Construction worker, waitress, farm worker:**

  250 cph x 8 hours = 2000 calories

ACTIVITY TIME

Work, travel and sleep make
up the usual daily routine of
most people. Activity time
normally associated with the
period after work and on the
weekends is when we can
make the largest contribution
to our daily calorie burn. If
we are involved in a non-
physical hobby, such as the
Internet, night school or
watching television, we will
add little to our daily calorie
burn total. If, on the other
hand, we go 'clubbing'
several times a week, belong
to a gym or play football on
the weekends, our overall
calorie burn will be
dramatically increased.

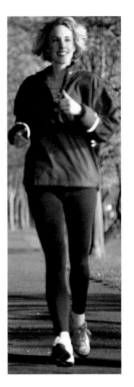

Raising the calorie burn
during some of our routine activities can also be
attained by short periods of greater activity. A good
example is walking all or part of the way to work, or
walking around the shops at lunchtime.

During any form of aerobic exercise, fat is only one
source of energy used by the body: it will also use
carbohydrates from any food consumed. This means
that it can take a great deal of exercise to burn up a
significant amount of calories. For example, it takes
about a mile of walking at a normal pace to use up

100 calories. If you consider that there are 3500 calories in one pound of fat, this means it would take 35 miles of running or walking to burn them off.

> **CALORIE BURNS**

- ➤ Watching television, Internet   80 cph
- ➤ Walking, dancing   250 cph
- ➤ Jogging, tennis, cycling   300 cph
- ➤ Running, football   400 cph
- ➤ Bergen hillwalking, squash   500 cph

FLUID INTAKE

Fluid intake is vital because all body functions use water, added to which water accounts for almost 60 per cent of our body composition. It should, however, be noted that fat cells hold the least amount of water, which means the fatter we are the less water our bodies contain and therefore excessive water loss will make little difference to body weight loss. Additionally, if we have a low water content then our body minerals will not dissolve properly throughout our circulation.

Thirst and hunger control our intake while the kidneys direct the bulk of body fluid output, thus our body's water supply is kept in balance. If we become overweight or continue to consume too much of the wrong food and drink then we suffer an imbalance. There is a tendency with most people to forget the importance of fluid intake and the benefits associated with drinking fresh water. In general we eat less of those foods with a high water content, such as fruit and vegetables, cooked rice or pasta, in favour of foods with a low water content, such as meat and sugars. Additionally, we tend to drink more tea, coffee, soft drinks and alcohol than we do fresh water, and so most people live with a water imbalance.

Fresh Clean Water

Drinking fresh water is just about the best thing you can drink to control the body's fluid balance. It will seem strange to begin with, but try replacing your daily cups of tea with water. At first you will find

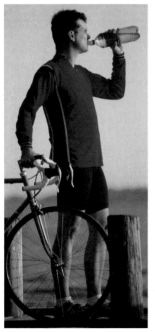

yourself drinking double the amount, which is good, and you will gain no weight. After the first few weeks your system will start to show the benefits, with a clearer complexion and a reduction in the amount of body pain encountered while exercising.

Depending on its source, water will differ in taste. Natural spring water is best and a large variety is available in all supermarkets. However, my advice is to do a little research at your local library and find out where the nearest natural spring is, then drive there and fill as many containers as possible. Consuming around three litres a day will result in a diminished craving for food and alcohol. It will aid sweating during exercise, making the skin healthier and the muscles supple.

DRINKING ALCOHOL

In addition to food and water most people consume varying amounts of alcohol. Due to alcohol's high calorific value, it has a significant effect on diet and fitness. As already mentioned, fat contains nine calories per gram, carbohydrates and protein contain four calories per gram but alcohol contains seven calories per gram.

Small amounts of alcohol drunk occasionally do little or no harm, and there are those who consider that small quantities are actually beneficial. By and large, drinking falls into two categories: drinking for pleasure or reward, or drinking to fulfil a dependency.

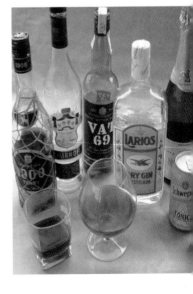

Drinking occasionally and in moderate amounts will have no effect on your physical fitness, but those with alcohol dependency put themselves at risk because exercising with a high blood alcohol content can cause death.

Spirits are absorbed quicker than beer, and fizzy mixers only help to speed up the process. Eating will slow down the rate at which alcohol is absorbed into the bloodstream, and the more weight we carry the longer it will take for alcohol to have any effect. As a rough guide the blood alcohol level per 100 ml of blood will be as follows.

➤ 1 pint of beer or 2 shots of spirit = 30 mg
➤ 2 pints of beer or 5 shots of spirit = 60 mg
➤ 5 pints of beer or 12 shots of spirit = 100 mg
➤ A bottle of spirits drunk within 4 hours = 400 mg

Even at 60 mg judgement can be defective and we start to lose discrimination and common sense. At 100 mg balance, vision and muscle control are all affected.

The point at which people switch from being a social drinker to one dependent on alcohol is a very grey area. For the most part people have an inbuilt regulator, and soon realize by their increasing number of hangovers and lack of concentration that they are drinking too much. The problem is further compounded by building up a tolerance to alcohol which means that increased amounts are required to achieve the same effect. This is the first sign that we are on the road to life-threatening alcohol dependency. In this event you are faced with one option – stop drinking.

Reduced Alcohol Intake

The relationship between alcohol and fitness is a balance, but quite simply the less you drink the fitter you are. If you drink too much alcohol then you need to bring your drinking under control. If you drink to excess, you will need to abstain altogether. If you drink socially, as most of us do, but feel you can control your drinking, you should still try to restrict the amount of alcohol you consume. You need only come up with a few reasonable excuses.

➤ I'm driving.

➤ I'm on prescribed drugs.

➤ I have a liver problem.

➤ I can't drink at lunchtime it makes me sleepy.

➤ Turn up late at parties and go home early.

➤ Drink mixers only and pretend they contain alcohol.

➤ Drink only every other day.

➤ Drink a glass of water between every alcoholic drink.

Go Dry

In the context of this book the only real option is abstinence. If you are only a social drinker then this will not be a problem. For those with a heavier consumption, it will do them the power of good to stop. The weight you lose when not drinking is a major bonus in itself.

SMOKING

We all know that smoking is bad for our health, but if

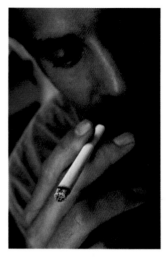

I were to say it interferes with physical fitness, I would be inundated with claims from very fit people who have always smoked. That said, I do urge those who smoke to give it up because smoking kills more than 100,000 people in Britain alone.

I have seen and listened to people who claim that they only smoke 5 cigarettes a day, and while there may be a few such people, the majority of smokers go through at least 20 cigarettes a day, such is the nature of the addiction.

Whatever the reasons for smoking – relaxation, stimulation, addiction – it seems to be one of the hardest habits to break, but it is reckoned that at least 40 per cent of smokers would give it up if they could. Millions are spent each years on one therapy after another by people trying to quit. Some do win through but many more fall by the wayside and continue smoking as before. There is only one way to give up smoking – willpower

Willpower

It is this ability which allows us to change our lives, and it is something that we all possess. Today I will try. If I fail then I will try again tomorrow. You may set your goal to quit smoking in the next two weeks, but even if it takes you two years you have still won.

You may think this is a non-smoker talking, but in fact, I used to smoke. The reason I stopped was simple: I wanted to get fit and without doubt, sticking to an aerobic fitness programme is one sure way of helping you quit smoking. The same motivation that gets you walking, running or working in the gym will help you deny your craving for a cigarette. The more you exercise the less you will smoke. Sustain your fitness programme and your willpower will increase.

STOPPING SMOKING

➤ Start a fitness aerobic programme.

➤ Tell everyone you are quitting - this puts pressure on you to do so.

➤ Find some activity that involves using your hands during period of relaxation.

➤ Remind yourself of the health benefits - longer and better life. You will get the opportunity to see your grandchildren.

➤ Think of the financial benefits. Not just the cost of the cigarettes but your pension. You will have paid all those contributions and not lived to receive a pension.

➤ Don't think you're a failureif during some social function you are seduced into smoking several cigarettes - quit again next day.

SLEEP

Sleeping is something we all do and need to do properly. It is an essential part of our lives especially when it comes to fitness and well-being. When we sleep, the whole body relaxes totally. Many people suffer from a poor night's sleep, or from not getting sufficient to refresh the body. On average most of us sleep for around 8 hours each night; however, it is quality rather than quantity which is important. Contrast waking after a restful night and feeling ready to take on the world with that of waking after a restless, short, or alcohol-induced sleep, wooly-headed and just as tired as when you went to bed. Lack of a good night's sleep not only results in loss of concentration and a poor work performance but it also has a very detrimental effect on health.

By far the largest single cause of sleeplessness is stress. This leads to insomnia which only acts to increase the stress starting a vicious circle which in extreme cases can cause a nervous breakdown. Stress is a major problem. If you fall asleep worrying, or lie awake with your mind constantly alert you are more than likely suffering from stress. Short-term worries, such as moving house, exam results, a business meeting, etc., are normal and pose no real problem. Long-term worries, however, for example a serious illness, death of a family member, redundancy or divorce, can all cause relentless insomnia.

In the normal course of events we should fall asleep within 15 minutes of getting into bed, but those suffering from acute insomnia may require some help.

Sleeping pills are useful for treating short-term sleep deprivation and in helping to restore a normal sleep pattern, but confronting and dealing with the underlying cause is the best approach.

NORMAL STAGES OF SLEEP

➤ Awake lying in bed resting for on average 15minutes.

➤ Blood pressure, heart rate and body temperature all fall.

➤ The mind drifts from consciousness to unconsciousness.

➤ After an hour or so the heart rate starts to increase as we start dreaming.

➤ We stop and start dreaming several times during the night.

➤ We wake.

The stage in which we dream is known as REM (rapid eye movement)sleep. These periods of REM sleep are essential to our well being, as their loss leads to aggressiveness and irritability. The taking of sleeping pills or other drugs and alcohol can interfere with REM sleep.

Getting a Good Nights Sleep

One of the best ways to promote sleep is to have a

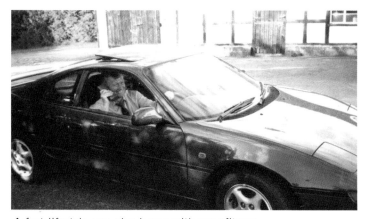

A fast lifestyle can play havoc with your fitness

good exercise routine. The fitter the body the better the sleep – no matter what worries you may have. Avoid having a nap during the day, as this may make it more difficult to get to sleep at night. Try to establish a pattern for your pre-sleep routine. Start winding down at least a couple of hours before your bedtime. Walk the dog, have a hot bath, watch the television or read a book – the important thing is to relax. Avoid eating late, or consuming too much alcohol just prior to going to bed. Milk contains trytophan which is a substance that helps you sleep, so make a milky drink before bedtime. If you wake in the night, don't drink coffee or tea, drink water instead

Midlife Crisis

I include this section to highlight a problem which affects many people and males in particular. Men do not have a sudden hormonal change like menopausal-women, but they do change. Most of that change is stress-related, bringing with it many problems and changes in behaviour. This change takes place anywhere between 35 and 45, depending on the individual, although the symptoms are usually the same for everyone. Factors such as overwork, fatigue, excessive intake of alcohol, heavy smoking and failing sex drive, all contribute to a downward spiral in general well-being.

Many married men suffering a midlife crisis turn to a younger woman hoping to rejuvenate their earlier masculinity. Those that do not stray, preferring to treat the midlife crisis as a fait accompli, follow an equally problematic path as their mood swings and sexual indifference can also have a dramatic affect on their partners. When a woman feels she no longer inspires affection or desire in her partner, she feels rejected, and continued feelings of rejection can lead to tension and squabbling. If not remedied, this escalates to affect the whole family.

Midlife Fitness

The answer is simple; reduce your stress load, alcohol consumption and smoking through fitness. This book is ideally suited to those suffering from a midlife crisis. Begin by seeing your doctor and having a general check-up. Then set your goal and aim to achieve it. Plan some surprise for your partner to coincide with the end of your fitness programme. Take your loved one on holiday and show off your new-found energy.

REMEMBER

➤ See your doctor for a check-up.

➤ Reduce your intake of alcohol.

➤ Lose weight if necessary.

➤ Plan an exercise programme.

➤ Be happy with what you have - not what you want.

Weight-loss Programme

The Weight-loss Programme is mainly aimed at those people (including myself) who are so far overweight that strenuous exercise is both impracticable and dangerous. This doesn't mean we cannot exercise, it simply means we must first correctly adjust our body weight. The programme also is an excellent guide for those who simply wish to lose weight. For those very overweight I suggest that you repeat this programme until you have achieved your desired goal.

To start with, be honest with yourself and define what stage you are at now, then set yourself a target. This means determining your body weight and fitness levels as well as examining your daily routine, both at work and at home. It also means taking a good look at your diet and lifestyle, such as drinking and keeping late nights. Another consideration prior to embarking on a weight-loss and fitness programme is your age – will your body stand it?

Exercise is only one part of the equation when it comes to getting fit: nutrition is just as important if the body is to perform at its maximum potential. The following chapter aims to set out the basic principles of nutrition and give guidance for achieving weight control and strengthening physical performance.

EATING HEALTHILY

In the UK and USA there is a great deal of talk about eating healthily but few people lead by example. However, this is not true of all nations. For example, in the Mediterranean countries most people eat a well-balanced diet, and the beneficial results are clear to see. I do not say that such eating habits are a 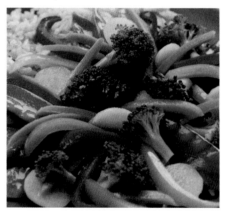 deliberate attempt to diet, more that circumstance and nature have provided a range of staple foods that are very healthy as well as being native to the region. Most of the Mediterranean coastal area is one large garden, producing a wide range of fruit and vegetables, olive oil and fish. The abundance of free spring water in most towns and villages and the added bonus of clean, dry air also undoubtedly help.

Lifestyle Eating

The way we eat and what we eat is directly related to our social circumstances and lifestyle. Some people will eat only fish and chips or beans on toast because that is all they can afford, while others will eat the same merely from habit or because it is the easiest option. At the other end of the scale, being in the position to buy expensive business lunches or indulge in exotic foods is no guarantee that you are providing your body with a well-balanced diet.

In addition to individual circumstances and lifestyle there is the added media pressure of what is good or bad for us, according to the latest research. 'Don't eat butter it's really bad for you.' 'Eggs will give you salmonella.' You may think it madness to ignore professional medical opinion but recently my mother recalled that as a young girl, between the wars, she had helped her granny make enormous breakfasts for the farmer husband and his workers. These included eggs, home-cured fat bacon, toast and lashings of home-made salty butter – and there was still lunch and the evening meal to go. It was a time when farming was still very labour intensive and farm workers worked long hours. Butter, full-cream milk, home-made bread all saturated with salt and fats were the mainstay diet of most of my fore-family, many of whom lived into their late nineties. My mother is now 80 years old and she still dances, goes shopping on her bike, has an active brain and frequently travels abroad. The point she was trying to make is: it's not what we eat, it's is how well our body converts the food energy we supply it with. Life today is much easier than it was in 1925. Our day-to-day physical workload is less demanding and to compensate we must live on a diet free of fat and dairy products in order to keep our cholesterol in check.

AUTHOR'S NOTE

➤ Before moving to Spain I tried several diets but they did little. I simply stayed the same weight or became heavier. But four months in Spain and I have lost three stone – why? Diet, fresh air, water and exercise in that order.

➤ The diet was not planned but just included local foods, mainly fresh fish, seafood and salads. Cooking was all done by grilling or with virgin olive oil; the latter was also mixed with a little vinegar to make the salad dressing. At least 90 per cent of the meals were cooked outdoors, barbecue style. Due to the heat most Spaniards spend a lot of their time sitting outdoors. The heat makes you sweat, and the need to slake your thirst is constant. There is local spring water freely available and a constant supply of fresh orange juice, either from the local trees or the supermarket. So I drank a great deal more of both than I used to. Also, keeping to the exercise programmes in this book encouraged me to walk the local mountain paths or go for a bike ride along the quiet roads, which became more of a pleasure than a chore.

➤ Despite this sounding like a promotion for everyone to live in Spain, the point I am

(contd)

trying to make is that these factors really do promote a healthier lifestyle and a natural loss of body weight.

OBESITY

Obesity poses a serious health risk. There is only one real answer to the problem and that is to lose weight. Other than surgery, the only way to achieve this is to consume fewer calories and steadily increase the amount of aerobic exercise taken. If you do not have the will-power to do this, then you may need to find a partner or join a diet organization. Even if you do join a group, you must still make time in your home life for regular exercise as this will help keep you on track when your group course has finished.

The advantages of reversing the effects of obesity are numerous – a slimmer more attractive figure, a fitter and more agile body and a better lifestyle overall. What must be kept in mind is the time span over which any weight loss should occur. Because someone who is obese is unable to participate in strenuous exercise, the initial weight loss will be achieved through diet. This involves keeping strict control over calorie intake while maintaining the body's nutritional requirements. How much we need to lose and over what period of time can be discovered by simple mathematical equations, shown overleaf.

BODY MASS INDEX (BMI)

BMI is defined as your weight in kilos divided by your height in metres squared. The recommended BMI in women is set between 18–23, while in men it is 21–26.

For example, for a woman who is 5 feet 6 inches tall and weighs 12 stone 5 lbs the calculation would be:

77.85 kilos ÷ 2.72 m (1.65 x 1.65) = 28.62

(to convert lbs to kilos multiply by 0.45; to convert inches to metres multiply by 0.025)

The upper BMI limit in women is 23, which when subtracted from 28.62 leaves 5.62. This figure multiplied by the height squared, 2.72, equals 15.28, which is the number of kilos she is overweight.

The recommended weight loss per week is 2.25 lbs (1 kilo), therefore it will take some 15 weeks for her to achieve her goal.

Another more simple way of assessing weight is to grab the skin at the side of your waist between your fingers and thumb without pulling. Measure the overhang of skin and estimate the depth. If its more than a centimetre thick you are carrying excess fat. To estimate the amount ignore the first 2.5 cm (1 inch) then multiply every centimetre over by 10 kg (22 lb). For example, if your skin pinch is 5 cm (2 inches) in total you will be roughly 25 kg (55 lb) overweight.

AUTHOR'S NOTE

➤ When I joined SAS Selection I had been working out with a bergen for several months and considered myself fit. When I arrived at Hereford it was plain to see that many candidates had not bothered to exercise and as a result most were dismissed in the first few days. Not all of the overweight candidates failed as some, who I would call borderline cases, seemed to have the determination to keep going. One such candidate passed selection and remained with the SAS for 15 years, during which time he always looked fat and overweight. Yet this did not affect his fitness or make him slow during exercise activities. Looking overweight doesn't necessarily mean you're unfit.

WEIGHT-LOSS REGULATION

Weight-loss and physical-training programmes for overweight people can only work through regular exercise and reduced calorie consumption. The type of exercise we undertake affects the amount and nature of the weight loss. Both running and walking burn about 100 calories per mile. One pound of fat contains 3500 calories. Thus, burning one pound of fat through exercise alone requires a great deal of running or walking. On the other hand, weight lost through dieting alone includes the loss of useful muscle tissue. Those who participate in an exercise programme that emphasizes the development of strength and muscular endurance, however, can actually increase their muscle mass while losing body fat. These facts help explain why exercise and good dietary practices must be combined.

It is possible to determine how much excess weight we are carrying and adjust our calorific requirements to safely and successfully lose excess fat. We can also devise a sound individualized exercise plan which will develop useful muscle tissue while increasing fat loss. Generally, overweight people should strive to reduce their fat weight by 2.25 lbs (1 kilo) per week.

However, it should be remembered that when we start to lose weight, either by diet or exercise or both, a large weight loss is not unusual. This may be due to water loss associated with the using up of the body's carbohydrate stores. Although these losses may be encouraging, little of this initial weight loss is due to the disappearance of fat. Weighing under similar circumstances and at the same time each day will accurately monitor progress. This helps avoid false measurements due to normal fluctuations in body weight during the day. As a person develops muscular endurance and strength, lean muscle mass generally increases. Because muscle weighs more per unit of volume than fat, caution is advised in assessing a person's weight loss progress. Just because a person is not losing weight rapidly does not necessarily mean they are not losing fat. In fact, a good fitness programme often results in gaining muscle mass while simultaneously losing fat weight. If there is reasonable doubt, the percentage of body fat should be determined and a revised fitness programme begun if need be.

One good idea is to keep a calorie control chart in your kitchen. As you prepare or eat food mark down the quantity and the calories. This will give you an understanding of the food value and help you regulate your diet. Fresh fruit need not be counted in this chart, but it should be considered as a perk. Likewise, the best way to monitor your progress is to get a calendar and fill in the weight each day. If you don't want anyone to know about your diet or see your progress keep it in a safe place.

ESTIMATING YOUR PRESENT CONDITION

For the purpose of this book it is argued that three overriding factors govern our lives: age, health and weight. If you are 22-years-old, of average height, with no illness and weigh around 11 stone (if you are a man) or 10 stone (if you are a woman) then you have no problem. If on the other hand you are 55-years-old, average height with a slight heart problem and weigh 16 stone, you need to think about weight loss before starting any serious exercise.

The following is a rough guide as to what you can expect from your body through different ages.

Aged 18–25

This is when the body is at its peak of fitness. Most people in this age group find natural fitness through a healthy social life. Dancing, late nights and an active sex life make for a high calorie burn.

26–36

This is the time when most people get married. A supply of steady work is required to protect the family interests, such as paying the mortgage and seeing to the family's needs. Stress can become a health factor. The body's fitness is still maintained by the demands of home-building.

36–45

The risk of heart disease starts to increase. This is the time when the body's calorific needs start to decline and the weight goes on. Daily alcohol intake may increase. This is an important time to review one's lifestyle. Fitness now needs constant attention and work – social sports, such as football and squash will help.

46–60

Heart disease is the main killer, but if you take up steady exercise again, it is possible to improve your lifestyle. Long walks, gardening, and a careful diet will help maintain your fitness.

60 plus

This is the stage where your previous lifestyle catches up with you. If you have abused your body then you will start to suffer now that you are older. If you have had a healthy life then there's no reason why you should not live to a ripe old age. Continue eating a healthy diet and take daily exercise.

PERSONAL ASSESSMENT

This is the moment of truth. If you have purchased this book and are serious about getting fit or losing weight then you must first assess your present condition. The best way to do this is to stand naked in front of the mirror and turn around slowly. Next, to confirm your worst fears, step onto the bathroom scales and weigh yourself. Then work out your excess fat using the BMI method on page 63 and compare the results with the Height to Weight Chart opposite. (Note: If you have a small frame then deduct $4\frac{1}{2}$ lbs (2 kg) from the range, if you have a large frame, add $4\frac{1}{2}$lbs (2 kg) to the range.)

WEIGHT TO HEIGHT CHART

Men		Women	
Height	Av. Frame	Height	Av. Frame
5' 4"	9-9.3 st	4' 11"	7.4-8.2 st
(1.62 m)	(56.5-62 kg)	(1.52 m)	(46-51.5 kg)
5' 5"	9.2-10 st	5' 1"	7.5-8.4 st
(1.65 m)	(57.5-63 kg)	(1.55 m)	(47-52.5 kg)
5' 6"	9.4-10.4 st	5' 2"	7.8-8.6 st
(1.68 m)	(59-65 kg)	(1.57 m)	(48.5-54 kg)
5' 7"	9.8-11 st	5' 3"	8-8.9 st
(1.70 m)	(61-69 kg)	(1.60 m)	(50-55.5 kg)

5′ 8″	10-11 st	5′ 4″	8.2-9.2 st
(1.72 m)	(62.5-69 kg)	(1.62 m)	(51.5-57 kg)
5′ 9″	10.3-11.3 st	5′ 5″	8.4-9.4 st
(1.75 m)	(64.5-71 kg)	(1.65 m)	(52.5-59 kg)
5′ 10″	10.3-11.3 st	5′ 6″	8.7-9.4 st
(1.78 m)	(66.5-72 kg)	(1.68 m)	(54.5-61 kg)
5′ 11″	10.6-11.5 st	5′ 7″	9-10.4 st
(1.80 m)	(68-75 kg)	(1.70 m)	(56.5-65 kg)
6′ 0″	10.9-12 st	5′ 8″	9.3-10.7 st
(1.83 m)	(70-77.5 kg)	(1.72 m)	(58-67 kg)
6′ 1″	11.2-12.4 st	5′ 9″	9.6-11 st
(1.85 m)	(72-79.5 kg)	(1.75 m)	(60-69 kg)
6′ 2″	11.5-12.7 st	5′ 10″	9.9-11.2 st
(1.88m)	(73.5-82 kg)	(1.78 m)	(62-70.5 kg)
6′ 3″	12.1-13.4 st	5′ 11″	10.1-11.5 st
(1.90m)	(76-84 kg)	(1.80 m)	(63.5-78 kg)
6′ 4″	12.5-13.8 st	6′ 0″	10.4-11.8 st
(1.93m)	(78-86.5 kg)	(1.83 m)	(65-73.5 kg)

DO YOU WEIGH TOO MUCH?

If you are within the BMI range and your weight and height fit in with the chart, give or take a few pounds, then you don't really need to follow the Weight-loss Programme and can proceed straight to Programme One (see p.93). For those who are half a stone (3.1kg) overweight, first get a checkup from your doctor to make sure you are fit enough to start exercising. Only then should you proceed to Prog-ramme One. If you are more than a stone over-weight, any exercise will carry the risk of serious injury as the added weight will impose extra strain on joints, and increase the already overworked organs such as your heart and lungs. Sudden, enforced exercise on an overweight body can lead to a heart attack. Consult your doctor and carry out the Weight-loss Programme first.

WARNING

➤ Do not conduct the following fitness test if you have recently suffered from any illness, have heart problems, are taking prescribed medication or have been drinking heavily within the past 24 hours. Check the following questions and seek qualified medical advice if the answer to any is 'yes':

➤ Do you suffer from heart problems?

➤ Do you have high blood pressure?

➤ Do you suffer from chest pains?

➤ Do you suffer from dizziness or regular headaches?

➤ Do you have a medical condition that prevents exercise?

➤ Are you on medication?

➤ Are you 30 years or older and new to fitness?

➤ Are you seriously overweight?

FITNESS TEST

Being of normal weight for your stature and height does not automatically mean you are fit, it simply means you are not carrying excess fat. Having established your weight you now need to determine your present standard of fitness. This is a simple process whereby you monitor your heartbeat both at rest and during a set activity.

Resting Heart Rate (RHR)

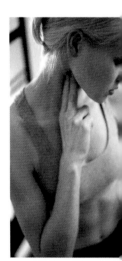

Sit quietly in a chair and relax for a full five minutes. Then check your pulse rate by placing two fingers on the carotid artery in your neck or on the inner wrist. Count the total number of beats for 30 seconds then double the number – this is your resting heart rate. The average is around 75 beats per minute. Slightly lower is excellent, but if your count is 85 or higher then you could have a problem.

Step Test

Find a step not less than 12 inches (30 cm) but not more than 16 inches (40cm) high. Start stepping up and down at a non-stop, steady rate for 5 minutes. Stop, sit in a resting position and take your pulse rate for 30 seconds, doubling the number to calculate for one minute. The average should be around 140 beats. Lower is good but any higher and you are unfit.

Blood Pressure

Go to your doctor or practice nurse and get your

blood pressure tested. Don't worry about being a pest as most surgeries encourage people to have a checkup. A normal person in their mid-thirties will have a blood pressure of around 120 over 80, but the doctor will indicate any risk if different.

HOW HARD CAN WE EXERCISE?

This is best answered by the individual in relation to their present weight and level of physical fitness. Exercising means working the body harder than normal but if you exercise to much too soon the body will rebel and it can be dangerous.

One of the best indicators of how our body is performing is heartbeat. If we are resting, the heart beats slower with a more relaxed rhythm, which is known as the *resting heart rate* (RHR). The harder we work the body the harder the heart works, but there is a limit known as the *maximum heart rate* (MHR). As a general rule you should exercise to around 70 to 75 per cent of your MHR, and this threshold is known as your *training heart rate* (THR).

To calculate your training heart rate you need to establish your RHR. For the purpose of this calculation we will assume that an average, healthy 25 year old not on medication has a RHR of 67. We must also determine our MHR which is done by subtracting our age from the number 220, i.e. 220 - 25 = 195. This means that our individual could exercise their heart to where it reaches a maximum of 195 beats per minute.

220 - age 25 = 195 maximum beats per minutes.

The difference between out resting heart rate and our maximum heart rate is our heart rate reserve (HRR). Calculated as follows, MHR - RHR = HRR.

195 - 67 = 128 beats per minute.

To find our training heart rate we simply calculate 70 per cent of the heart rate reserve and add it to our resting heart rate. Calculated as follows, 70 per cent of HRR + RHR = THR.

0.70 x 128 + 67 = 156.6

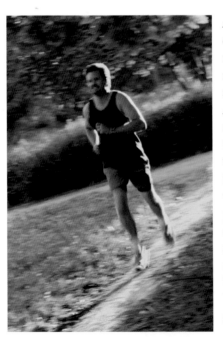

As the body is exercised the heat rate increases, the muscles produce heat and the body warms. After several minutes and depending on the exercise the body will settle and the increased heart rate will level off. After a period of 20 minutes check your heart rate and make this as accurate as possible by counting the pulse beats for at least 30 seconds. If you find

that your heart rate has jumped to more than your
training heart rate, you should reduce exercise intensity, likewise if it is below you should increase exercise
intensity.

The Mechanism Governing Fitness

What is physical fitness? Physical fitness gives us the
capability to function efficiently while at work or at
play. The main mechanisms of involved with physical
fitness are:

➤ Body Composition. (We cannot exercise properly
if our body is grossly overweight)

➤ Flexibility. (We cannot move freely if our body is
inflexible)

➤ Cardio respiratory endurance and efficiency.
(We cannot run if our body cannot breath)

➤ Muscular strength and endurance. (We can not
function without muscle strength)

BEST 10 EXERCISE ACTIVITIES (BY PERCENTAGE)

	Aerobic	Muscle	Flexibility
Running	100	90	30
Cycling	100	90	60
Weightlifting	20	100	80
Hillwalking	80	100	80
Step-ups	80	50	70

Badminton	60	60	60
Gymnastics	20	90	100
Walking	60	30	20
Squash	60	70	90
Gardening	60	60	60

PRINCIPLES OF EXERCISE

Before we exercise we must first of all set ourselves a goal, which can be established by asking why we are exercising; for example, it may be to run a marathon or to lose weight. The next thing is to make sure you are capable of achieving this goal and if not, why not and what can you do about it. People only get fit if they stick to the basic principles of exercise and diet. These basic principles apply to everyone irrespective of present levels of physical fitness.

➤ You should find the right balance between diet and fitness. No beginner who is overweight should start any strenuous exercise until their weigh has been reduced to a safe level. Likewise, for the more advanced, there is a need to balance the body's calorie intake against that consumed by disproportionate exercise.

➤ You must exercise on a regular basis. Exercise should be no different to sleep or work it is a function that we must do as a matter of course.

Ideally you should workout for a minimum of 3 periods per week up to a maximum of 5 periods per week.

➤ Any physical exercise should be progression. You should start off with less strenuous exercises for a short amount of time slowly building the intensity and duration. Your body will only become fitter when the workload of each exercise session exceeds that normally used by daily living demands.

STAGES OF ADVANCEMENT

It is not a good idea to go straight into a gym and begin serious weight exercises. First you must regulate your weight, after which you are better advised to attain a good level of aerobic fitness. Always start and finish your workout with a simple set of flexibility exercises suitable to your main activity. Your main activities should also be progressive, i.e. walking, jogging and then running. As you progress, take stock of your body, those who feel breathless or whose heart rate rises beyond their training heart rate while running should resume walking until the heart rate returns to the correct training level. Likewise where the route has a severe incline reduce your pace or walk. Once you can run for 30 minutes at a reasonable pace without breathing or muscle problems you can progress to resistance/weight training. No mater what programme you follow you must give the body time to recover, an exercise-free day between each

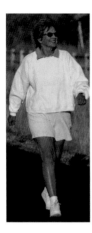
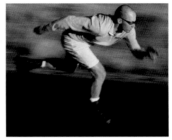
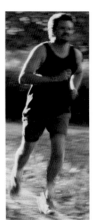

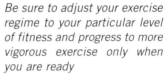
Be sure to adjust your exercise regime to your particular level of fitness and progress to more vigorous exercise only when you are ready

workout is normally long enough. Those who wish to train on a daily basis should alternate their workouts, e.g. one day in the gym and one day on the road.

To reach the desired level of fitness, you must increase the amount of exercise and/or the workout intensity as your strength and endurance increases. To improve cardio-respiratory endurance you must increase the length of time you run. For weight training you need to increase the resistance and number of sets per exercise.

Your diet and physical training should put emphasis on progressive conditioning of the whole body. Even though exercise is the key to sensible weight loss, reducing the number of calories consumed is equally important, although weight lost through dieting alone includes the loss of useful muscle tissue.

The type of exercise undertaken reflects on the

amount and nature of the weight loss. Those who participate in an exercise programme that emphasizes the development of strength and muscular endurance, however, can actually increase their muscle mass while losing body fat.

Stages of Attaining Fitness

As mentioned at the start, attaining a required level of fitness depends on present body composition, flexibility, cardio-respiratory exercise together with improved muscle strength and endurance. Prolonged physical fitness increases the efficiency of the heart and lungs, which help to deliver oxygen and nutrients needed for muscular activity. Muscular strength is also improved, allowing muscle groups to be exerted for a longer period. The ability to move the joints or any group of joints with a greater degree of flexibility through a normal range of motions becomes easier while body fat is depleted.

There are several types of fitness, including aerobic, anaerobic, isometric and isokinetic. The range of exercises involved in fitness varies from walking (aerobic) through to using weight machines in a gym (isokinetic). Although all are beneficial, the aim of this book is to concentrate primarily on aerobic and muscular fitness through simple exercises such as walking, running and hillwalking with a bergen (rucksack), following a similar structure to that of SAS Selection.

Likewise, this book is based on a long-term (six-month) diet and exercise routine, the idea being for you to attain the correct body weight before moving on to more progressive cardio-respiratory and muscle-resistance exercises. Once this has been achieved, you can then move on to tackle some serious fitness work. The range of weight-loss and physical exercises featured is fairly diverse but those chosen are simple, work extremely well and require the minimum of equipment.

TRAINING DAYS

One of the biggest factors that stop people doing any form of fitness training is the establishment of the daily work practise and/or home-life routine. For example, a junior doctor may work a 24-hour shift in a highly stressful environment, relishing the moment they can get to bed. Such a routine offers little chance of participating in any fitness programme. By contrast a professional soldier is encouraged to do at least an hour of fitness training every day with at least one afternoon given over to participation in a particular sport.

For most people the working week consists of Monday to Friday with the weekend relatively free. I say relatively because apart from work there are always important chores to do around the home as well as family commitments. The working day normally offers three periods for fitness training; before work, lunchtime and after work.

➤   Before work is the best option but this requires an early rise. However, it will give you more energy during your working day.

➤ Lunch time training is not really a good idea because for most people this has a tendency to be rushed resulting in little if any physical benefit.

➤ After work training normally provides more time but you are exercising after a full days work which can result in less than your best effort.

Weekends although free from your usual work routine have a nasty habit of building up jobs that cannot be completed during the working week. These include quality time with your partner and or children, shopping, plus home and car maintenance, and so on. However, both Saturday and Sunday are a more relaxing time and it is always possible to make time for additional exercise.

If you are starting your fitness programme from scratch you might also consider waiting until you have a break from work or a holiday. Such a period is ideal for starting a fitness programme and helping you structure a routine that can be sustained when you go back to work.

SELECTING THE RIGHT RUNNING SHOE

Running Shoes

I have lost count of the number of running shoes I have purchased over the years. During my service in the SAS the attrition rate meant a new pair very four to six months. The difference in shoes was quite amazing, while most would fit well enough the structure and therefore reaction on my feet while running varied enormously. It took me several years to realize that I had loose-jointed feet and that I require a firm fitting shoe in order to control the give when my feet made contact with the ground. Once I realized this I found I could run with a much easier and steadier pace, greatly reducing the hammering I had been giving my legs muscles and lower back.

RUNNING SHOES

➤ Never listen to the advertising claims.

➤ Choose a shoe for training not for racing.

➤ Make sure the fits snugly all over the foot without any pinching spots.

➤ Wear socks similar to those you train in when trying on you new shoes.

➤ Always try on both shoes and check the shoes for defects.

Checking your Feet

There are several simple ways to check out your feet and running shoes. The first one is to remove your shoes and socks and stand with your feet in a bowl of water, now step out and make an imprint on a flat surface such as the tiles on a bathroom floor. Check the shape of the foot imprint:

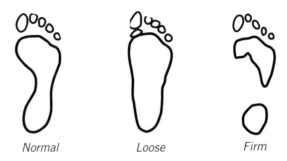

Normal   Loose   Firm

Next check an old pair of training shoes and look for signs of wear on the sole (the dark areas in the diagrams below) and on the heels.

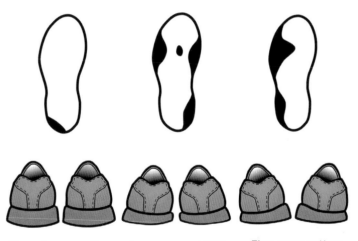

Normal wear pattern   Loose wear pattern   Firm wear pattern

Loose Feet

Running in the wrong show with loose feet can cause instability, leading to injuries at the heel, ankle and knee.

Firm Feet

Running in the wrong shoe with firm feet cause impact injuries. Pressure is pushed from the toes affecting all parts of the foot, leg and hips.

Eight-week Two-Stone Weight-loss Routine

The following weight-loss programme consists of diet and light exercise. Its purpose is to reduce body weight to the point where strenuous physical exercise will cause no harm or undue strain on bone or muscles. The programme will work best if you incorporate it into your daily life. The foods listed below are only a guide, you may select different foods as long as they contain roughly the same calorie count and you include a wide variety to ensure you get all the necessary nutrients. Keeping a daily calorie intake and weight log are essential.

This eight-week weight-loss routine is designed to reduce your calorie intake while gently getting your heart and lungs pumping and your muscles working. The diet is not excessive, just choose any one of the seven choices or similar for each of your three daily meals. You may have the same meals twice in the same week if you so wish. The breakfasts and lunches are straightforward but follow the instructions for preparing the dinner menus in the chapter on diet. Again, providing the calorie count is similar, you may devise your own meals (a list of foods and their calorific values can be found at the end of this book).

The physical workout is not difficult and consists mainly of walking, step-ups and sit-ups. The programme can be completed in 30 minutes and should be carried out in the morning and early evening. Where possible they should be incorporated into your daily routine.

GROUND RULES

➤ Calorie count all your meals. Maximum 1500 calories per day for men, 1300 for women.

➤ No eating or snacks after 6pm in the evening (water consumption only).

➤ No alcohol for the first week and then mid-week only thereafter; maximum of five measures over the weekend. Avoid spirits if at all possible.

➤ Drink at least two litres of water per day.

➤ Eat at least two pieces of fruit a day.

➤ Prepare and cook fresh food whenever possible.

➤ Don't skip an exercise because of the weather.

SAMPLE BREAKFASTS

One boiled or poached egg on one slice of toast
Bowl of cereal with fresh fruit and skimmed milk
Toast spread with either Marmite or honey
Bowl of fresh mixed fruit
Half tin of beans on toast

Half a honey-dew melon
Yoghurt

SAMPLE LUNCHES

Vegetable sandwich: beetroot, cucumber, tomato, lettuce,
cold potato
Home-made soup
Fresh fruit

SAMPLE DINNERS

Tuna or boiled egg salad
Cauliflower cheese with plain rice
Fitness Stew (see page xxx)
Whole trout with salad
Liver casserole
Slice of tortilla (Spanish omelette) and salad
Sausages and mash

SOFT DRINKS

Drink as much water as you like (spring water is best). Add a
small amount of Ribena or similar to add appeal if you find it
bland.

Pure orange juice from the supermarket is fine but freshly
squeezed is nutritionally better. Half a glass per day
maximum.

One glass per day of skimmed milk, including what you use
on your cereal.

No alcohol for the first week then limit yourself to a small amount each evening. Avoid all spirits and drink low-alcohol long drinks such as beer and cider. They will quench your thirst and your compulsion. No lunchtime drinking allowed.

LIGHT EXERCISES

As well as the diet it is important to start exercising. This will not involve anything strenuous but will help start to develop muscle tone and get you ready for a regular fitness routine. You should complete two sessions, one in the morning and one in the evening. Always relax before you start and let any food to digest for at least an hour. The walks and steps required during the first four weeks are purely to get you moving. Any set of steps inside or outside your home will suffice. The walks should always start and end at your front door and have a purpose if possible, such as going to the shops or walking the dog. Keep the walks as flat as possible and if you must walk uphill, do so slowly.

WARNING

➤   If, due to your weight, you are unable to carry out these two simple exercises then you should seek medical attention.

Walking

For most of us this natural exercise accounts for most of our daily calorie burn. For this reason those who walk or move around on their feet all day will generally be a lot fitter, such as a postman or nurse. The average person carrying no load should be able to walk at a pace of around 3.5 miles per hour over flat ground. According to your abilities, start off by walking at a slow pace, increasing speed and stride as your body gets warmer. You do not have to make a special effort to maintain a walking routine, it can become part of your daily travelling, for example, walking to and from work, or walking to the shops instead of taking the car.

The premise of this whole book is based on walking and as the weeks go by you will be able to increase your duration and start to walk over the cuntryside and hilly terrain (see Programme Two, p. 149). Building on this, you will eventually be able to walk some 12 miles (20 kilometres) over the mountains carrying a heavy rucksack.

Step-ups

Just like walking, most of us climb one or two sets of stairs during the day. This is an excellent form of aerobic exercise, but you should start off slow and build up carefully. Of all the aerobic exercises, steps are about the most beneficial while your body is overweight. The number of steps you need to exercise on can vary from 1 to 100, although a set of 10 is just about perfect, just walk up and down normally. However, doing step-ups for exercise does not require

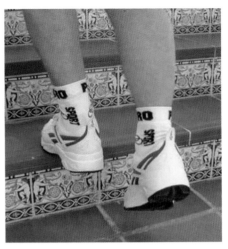

a flight of stairs as one step between 10–12 inches (25–30 cm) high will suffice. This can be a bench, concrete block or door step. The exercise is easy: step-up one foot after the other, then step down and repeat. Whatever number you climb the initial pace should be set at 50 steps per minute, descents not included. For example, if you have 10 steps in your flight you will need to climb and descend them 6 times in a minute. Increase the number and speed of the steps you do in a session, as you feel able. Step-ups help strengthen the calf and thigh muscles.

Sit-ups

For those who wish to lose weight sit-ups are probably the best form of exercise because they improve the strength of the abdominal muscles. As with other exercises there are many varieties, but for the benefit of this book we will stick to two methods.

Lie down flat on the floor. Place your palms over your ears, with your elbows running parallel down your chest. Raise the head and shoulders together until the upper arm is resting on your chest (placing your hands behind your head increases the risk of damaging your neck and back muscles); relax and repeat the movement. Try to avoid getting into a 'rocking motion' as this reduces the efficiency of the exercise.

A far easier way to benefit from sit-ups is to purchase a purpose-built abdominal exerciser. These are little more than a support for the neck and shoulders because the weight is lifted by your hands pulling on a rocker-type bar. With this apparatus the number of sit-ups can be greatly increased without putting undue strain on the neck and back. Although these abdominal exercises will not reduce your weight by any significant amount they will firm up the muscles, making you look slimmer and thus feel better.

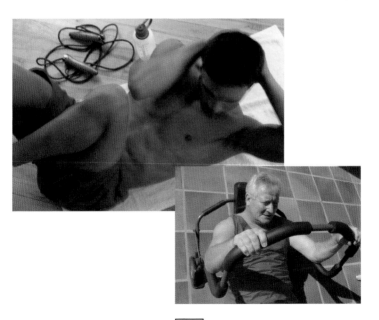

FIRST MONTH

Week 1 – exercise everyday

Morning: *Evening:*
2 x 50 steps in 2 min.   Repeat morning exercise
Rest
1-mile walk

Week 2 – exercise 6 days, rest 1

Morning: *Evening:*
3 x 60 steps in 3 min.   Repeat morning exercise
Rest
2-mile walk

Week 3 – exercise 6 days, rest 1

Morning: *Evening:*
4 x 70 steps in 4 min.   Repeat morning exercise
Rest
3-mile walk

Week 4 – exercise 6 days, rest 1

Morning: *Evening:*
5 x 80 steps in 5 min.   Repeat morning exercise
Rest
4-mile walk

SECOND MONTH

Week 1 – exercise 6 days, rest 1

Morning: *Evening:*
5 x 80 steps in 5 min.   Repeat morning exercise
Rest; 2 x 20 sit-ups;
Rest; 2 x 20 press-ups;
4-mile walk

Week 2 – exercise 6 days, rest 1
Morning: *Evening:*
5 x 80 steps in 5 min.   Rest
Rest; 3 x 20 sit-ups;
Rest; 3 x 20 press-ups;
4-mile walk

Week 3 – exercise 5 days, rest 2
Morning: *Evening:*
5 x 80 steps in 5 min.   5-mile walk
Rest; 4 x 20 sit-ups;
Rest; 4 x 20 press-ups;
5-mile walk

Week 4 – exercise 5 days, rest 2
Morning: *Evening:*
5 x 80 steps in 5 min.   Repeat morning exercise
Rest; 5 x 20 sit-ups;
Rest; 5 x 20 press-ups;
5-mile walk

By the end of the two-month programme you should be doing 4000 step-ups, 1000 sit-ups, 1000 press-ups and walking 50 miles per week. This equates to a calorie burn of around 7000 calories or 2 lbs of fat. If, in addition, you stick to the above diet for the two months you will lose at least two stone in weight. To reduce your weight further simply repeat week four of the second month.

Programme One

GETTING FIT

If you have managed to comply with the Weight-loss
Programme, or were one of those fortunate people
who were the correct weight to begin with, it is now
time to start getting fit. By completing the Weight-loss
Programme, or at least by staying within 80 per cent
of it, you will have accomplished several important
things. You will have achieved the discipline of a
regular routine and from here on in exercise will get
easier and become more enjoyable. Providing you
have stuck to the dietary requirements, you will have
flushed your system with water and reduced your
dependency on alcohol. Your breathing should be
easier, making your muscles more active which in turn
will add to your feel-good factor. But your main
reward will be when you step on the scales. If adhered
to correctly for the full twelve weeks, the programme
will produce a body weight loss of 20–24 lbs (9–11
kg).

If you are new to exercise, or have just finished the
Weight-loss Programme, set your exercise goal at
around 50 per cent of what you would like to achieve
for the first few months. As your heart rate and
breathing improve increase your goal to 75 per cent.

If you are still overweight then continue repeating the last week of weight-loss exercises until you reach your target weight, then move on to Programme One.

AUTHOR'S NOTE

➤ I am now one month into writing this book and have kept to the strict diet and exercise programme detailed in the Weight-loss Programme. The feel-good factor hit me when I weighed myself and found that my weight had fallen from 16st 7 lbs (105 kg) to 15st 11lbs (100 kg) – a loss of 10 lbs (4.5 kg). I checked the scales for several days after and my weight fluctuated no more than a couple of pounds either way. As I looked in the mirror I promised myself that by next month I would crack the 14-stone barrier. The problem remaining is one of bodyweight: I am still too heavy to start strenuous exercise. I am repeating the Weight-loss Programme for another month with the addition of two sets of floor exercises, which are designed to increase muscle strength and improve flexibility. What pleases me about the Weight-loss Programme is the fact that I do not feel as if I have deprived myself of any food – I have simply taken control of what goes in my mouth. severe arthritis in both my elbows

(contd)

and forearms, something I have endured since I was 30 years old. Over the past six months having replaced my tea drinking with water, the arthritic pain has all but disappeared. Whether this is down to my increased water intake I cannot say, but my gut feeling tells me it is.

Before we start our first exercise programme there are a few things to understand. These are fairly simple rules which will help guide and maintain your progress. In addition, you need to understand how to carry out each exercise properly and for the right duration.

GENERAL FITNESS RULES

➤ The two most important rules are: to set aside time for exercise and so build it into your lifestyle; to maintain a regular routine you must avoid injury, the chances of which can be reduced by warm-up exercises (see p.98).

MAINTAINING CALORIE INTAKE

For those people who have completed the Weight-loss Programme, remember to stay within the height-to-weight guidelines (see pp.67–68). Remember, your calorie intake can rise to help balance the energy output as you increase your amount of physical exercise.

The Amount of Calories You Need

To find out the amount of calories required to maintain your ideal weight convert your ideal body weight to pounds and multiply by 15 – this will give you your daily calorie intake. This is based on a moderately active person; those who do less exercise or physical work will require less and vice versa. For example, a nurse of medium build weighing 9st 2 lbs will require 1920 calories per day (128 lbs x 15) to maintain her ideal weight.

FREQUENCY OF TRAINING

It is the frequency of training which determines how fit you will become and how long you remain fit. The more exercise you do the fitter you will become until you reach your peak, or desired goal. This programme starts off by exercising every other day for periods of around one hour. After three weeks this is increased to five times a week with two rest days evenly spaced. There is also an increase in the duration of each session to around 90 minutes.

Once your fitness goal has been achieved you may wish to advance to a higher degree of fitness, or choose to switch to a more social form of exercise, such as squash. Frequency of training is best recorded in your weight and fitness log. This means you can keep a check on your progress and so help prevent you slipping back into old habits.

FLEXIBILITY

Another vital element of physical fitness is flexibility. Flexibility is the range of movement of a joint or series of joints and their associated muscles. Good flexibility can help you complete such physical tasks as lifting, loading, climbing, walking running, and swimming etc, with greater efficiency and less risk of injury. The body can flex its muscles in a multitude of directions, although there is no real test to determine the body's overall flexibility. The best way is to test flexibility is to assess the strain on the ham-string and low-back areas. These areas are vulnerable to injury in most people, mainly due to loss of flexibility. A simple

toe-touch test can be used - stand with your legs straight and feet together and bend forward slowly at the waist - if you cannot touch your toes without vigorous bending then you need to improve your flexibility.

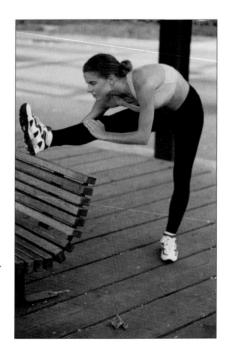

The best time to do stretching exercises is during your warm-up and cool down periods. The muscle should be stretched to full tension and a little beyond their normal capacity, causing strain but no pain. The range of stretching exercises varies from a gradual lengthening of the muscles as the body part moves around a joint to partner assisted stretching and muscle bouncing. For example a slow rotation of the arms through their full range will help increase joint mobility and loosen-up the surround muscle while jogging or walking on the spot for two minutes causes a steady raise in the heart rate, blood pressure and muscle temperature. Ideally, those stretching exercises used during a warm-up period should be held for around 10 seconds, while during the cool-down period the same exercise can be held for up to 20 seconds. The longer a stretch is held, the easier it is for the muscle to adapt to that length.

The type of flexibility exercise used should reflect on the muscle groups used during your main exercise period. If your main activity is a 5 mile run then your flexibility exercises should include thigh and hamstring flexing. If on the other hand you intend to do as session of muscular fitness then you flexibility exercises should mimic those activities: for example chest and abdominal flexing which helps prepare the neuromuscular pathways.

WARM-UP AND COOL-DOWN EXERCISES

Warm-up exercises increase body temperature. They also increase the range of joint movements and improve the speed of muscular contractions. In all the warm-up prepares the body in order that it will function throughout an energetic workout without injury.

By contrast many people do not understand the importance of cooling -down after strenuous exercise. Cooling down exercises bring the body back to its resting state in a measured way. To stop suddenly without any clod down exercise will cause blood to remain in the muscles thereby temporarily reducing the flow to the heart and brain. Feeling dizzy and faint directly after stopping any vigorous are sure signs of this.

1   Start by deep breathing, fully exhale, then inhale slowly to a count of 10
2   Exhale to a count of 10
3   Repeat this three times

The purpose of this is to increase the amount of oxygen being delivered to the muscles, which in turn produce energy. Deep breathing will also help you relax and make your body go loose.

Most warm-up exercises are simple rotation and have been around for many years. Rotation exercises are used to encourage joint lubrication and gently stretch the tendons, ligaments, and muscles associated with a joint. Depending on how you feel, spend around 30 seconds to a minute on each exercise. Start off gently, working all your muscles through the full extent of their function, speed up slightly as your heart rate increases.

The following are common stretching exercises which must be completed slowly before you undertake any rigorous activity.

Neck & Shoulders

Pose: Stand straight with your feet shoulder width apart. Place you hands on your hips.
Exercise: Roll the head in a loop 3 times around the shoulders ; repeat in the opposite direction.

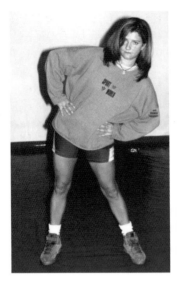

Method 2

Pose: Stand with your feet shoulder length apart with your arms behind your back griping your right wrist.
Exercise: Pull the right arm while twisting your head to look along the right shoulder. Do 5 repetitions then hold it for 10 seconds. Repeat with your left arm.

Arms & Shoulders

Pose: Stand straight with your feet shoulder width apart. Cross your arms at chest height.
Exercise: Swing each arm out in turn until it is extended at shoulder height. Return the arm the chest position. Repeat with the other arm. Do 10 alternate repetitions with each arm.

Method 2

Pose: Stand with your feet shoulder width apart. Extend your arms outward parallel to your shoulders.
Exercise: With arms out at 90 degrees from the body,

rotate the arms in a small circle for 10 repetitions. Reverse for 10 repetitions.

Chest

Pose: Stand straight with your feet shoulder length apart and your hands linked in the at-ease position behind your back.

Exercise: Lean forward forcing your arms up as high as possible, then bend your knees until you feel the chest expand. Hold this position for 10 seconds - repeat twice.

Method 2 (partner assisted)

Pose: Sit on the ground with your legs crossed and your arms outstretched. Your partner should stand behind you gripping your wrists.

Exercise: keep you head and back straight while your partner pulls back your expended arms to the point where there is mild discomfort. Hold for 15 seconds.

Trunk & Hips

Pose: Stand straight with your feet wide apart with right foot slight forward. Place your hands on your hips.

Exercise: Dip from the upright position to your right side without bending the trunk - 10 repetitions. Adopt the opposite position by extending your left foot and repeat the exercise.

Method 2

Pose: Stand straight with your feet shoulder width apart and stretch your arms into the air above your head.

Exercise: Without bending your knees, bring your arms down in front of you between your legs, and touch your toes. Return to the upright position, 10 repetitions.

Groin

Pose: Lunge forward bending your left knee while keeping the right leg straight. Balance by using your hands to grip your left knee.

Exercise: Stretch your body as far as possible over your left knee and hold for 15 seconds. Repeat using the opposite leg.

Method 2 (partner assisted)

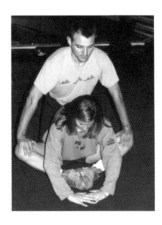

Pose: sit on the ground with you knees bent out and the soles of your feet together. The partner should kneel (with both legs) behind you.

Exercise: Lean forward, while your partner presses downwards on your inner knees. The pressure should cause slight discomfort. Hold the position for 15 seconds.

Thigh & Legs

Pose: Lie down flat on your stomach.
Exercise: Kick up your left leg and grip the toes with your right hand. Pull the foot into towards the buttock. Hold this position for 15 seconds. Repeat using the opposite leg. This exercise can also be done standing while balanced against a wall.

Method 2

Pose: Stand with your feet together arms at your side.
Exercise: Raise one leg gripping the knee with you hands and hugging it to your chest. Pull for about 15 seconds. Return to the rest position and repeat using the other leg.

Method 3

Pose: Find a wall or a tree and rest your palms flat against it. Open your legs to your normal stride, keeping your feet flat on the ground.
Exercise: Bend your right knee so that the calf muscle of the left leg (trailing leg) is lightly stretched. Hold for 10 seconds and switch legs. Repeat 3 times each leg.

Knees & Ankles

Pose: Stand with your feet together, slightly bent at the waist so that your hands rest on your knees.
Exercise: Keeping your feet steady, rotate you knees in a circular motion. 5 repetitions in each direction.

Hamstring

Pose: Sit on the floor with both legs fully extended

and slightly apart. Lean forward and grip your toes. **Exercise:** keep your back and head as straight as possible and lean back pulling on your toes.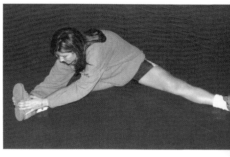

Hold the position for 10 seconds. Repeat 3 times.

Exercise Partners

For many of us, losing weight starts off as a very personal thing due mainly to our public declaration that we are unfit or overweight. While you may wish to exercise alone, you will achieve far better results if you choose to exercise with one or more partners.

The advantages are enormous, none more so than the maintenance of motivation. When you feel like giving up, your partner should impel you into continuing, and vice versa. Additionally, a common bond will develop that makes the routine more of a social pleasure than an individual endeavour. Some of the rewards of having good partners are:

➤   Shared motivation
➤   Good reliance on routine
➤   Stricter weight control
➤   Reduced exercise boredom
➤   Reduction in stress levels

> **EASY LISTENING**

➤ Listening to music or an instructional tape is a great way of taking your mind off the monotony of your morning jog or exercise routine. However, it does present several dangers. First off, running on a public highway while listening through a headset prevents you from hearing the traffic. Switch off and remove the headset wherever vehicles or moving machinery are present. Second, beware of the dangers of trying to stay in time with music or video exercises which have a fast beat.

CARDIO-RESPIRATORY EXERCISES

An aerobic exercise is one which is sustained steadily for a duration of time. Typical examples of such exercise are walking, running and swimming. These activities steadily increase the intake of air through the lungs while breathing. Anaerobic exercise, on the other hand, involves short bursts of activity, for example, tennis and football. These activities mainly use the oxygen which is stored in the muscles. In this book, for the most part, we will concentrate on aerobic fitness, which is aimed at increasing the heart rate. This increased heart rate, if sustained for 45 minutes or more, helps prompt the heart to grow more muscle, therefore next time we exercise we should find it marginally easier. A continuation of this process is known as 'physical fitness'. The body's cardiovascular and respiratory systems function together, especially during exercise or work, to ensure that adequate oxygen is supplied to the working muscles to produce energy for muscular contraction. When muscle activity is sustained they become tired. The point at which this tiredness occurs is relative to the oxygen circulating in the system. A high level of cardio-respiratory fitness permits continuous physical activity without a decline in performance and allows for rapid recovery following fatiguing physical activity. The more popular activities include:

➤ Non-apparatus exercise such as sit-ups etc.

➤ Step-ups

➤ Walking

➤ Jogging

➤ Running

➤ Skipping

➤ Cycling

These exercises ensure a greater amount of air passes through the lungs. The same exercise also increases the pumping action of the heart, helping transmit the oxygenated blood to the working muscle. This same heart action accelerates the return of veinous blood back to the heart were it is expelled via the lungs through increased breathing.

SAS FITNESS DEFINITIONS

Different exercises, varying stages of fitness, and terrain all demand modification in the amount of effort put into the overall workout. For example some exercises which involve walking or running over rough terrain will physically be more demanding than doing the same exercise on a flat road. Simple aerobic exercise raises your heart rate, increases oxygen intake and improves blood flow. It will tone muscle and reduce body fat.

However, you must exercise to suit your body weight; the heavier you are the slower you should perform. After a while, the more weight you lose the faster you can go. The reason for this is simply to avoid injury. These differentials are best described as follows:

Pace

➤ Walking pace should average 18 minutes per mile.

➤ Jogging pace should be around 12–15 minutes per mile.

➤ Slow Running 10 minutes per mile.

➤ Normal Running 8 minutes per mile.

➤ Short fast run 5–6 minutes per mile.

Normal Rate

Run at the same pace making sure you can maintain a steady rhythm to your breathing. This should be about 70–80 per cent of best-effort pace.

Best Effort

Best effort means just that, giving it 100 per cent plus. Always make sure that you have warmed up properly before starting out on a best-effort run, and that you cool down after. As with all the exercise tasks, start off at a good but controllable pace, speed up and then push yourself to the limit for the final third.

Jogging

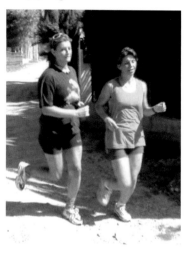

Jogging is little more than fast walking and the secret of jogging is duration, not speed. Time on your feet is what's important. Start your jogging programme only after two weeks of walking, especially if you are new to fitness. Once you start jogging, concentrate on a pace that suits you. Jog with a heel first action, letting the toes claw into the pace and push off with the ball of your foot. Jog within your breathing capabilities, that is, run at a pace where you can hold a normal conversation.

Running

It may sound silly but many people have forgotten or don't know how to run properly. The first thing to do is make sure your footwear is suited to the terrain you will be covering; blisters can be extremely painful (see Boots and Footwear, p. xxx).

Run with your body in an upright relaxed posture and let your arms adopt a natural swinging motion between your waist and chest. Run lightly making sure that your footstrike hits the ground with rhythmic timing. Shorten your step on the incline and extend it slightly on the decline. If your route takes you over uneven ground, be careful to avoid stepping on loose or protruding objects. Don't run too fast; you should be able to talk while running.

The terrain over which you run should also be considered. Remember we are not trying for Selection, so there is no need to take a dangerous route over rocky or marshy ground. Choose your route for its even pathways, its scenic beauty and its ease of access. If the route has very steep inclines then vary your pace accordingly.

March

The SAS terminology for walking with a bergen over the hills. Try to maintain a steady pace, walking all the time. Don't be tempted to run downhill during your build-up training - it is the easiest way to injure yourself.

Orienteering

Running at normal pace while following a set route around given points. It is used to develop map and compass skills. Introduce this type of training into your programme at the earliest opportunity.

Repetition Training

Run over level ground at your best effort for 1 minute, then jog for one minute. Start by doing this 3 times, building up to 6 of each. Once you can run and jog comfortably for 1-minute intervals, increase the distance to 90 seconds and so on.

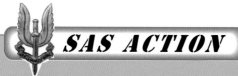

SAS ACTION

➤ During SAS Selection, I found that the best way to face a route was to split it into quarters. For the first quarter I would go slow, getting used to the bergen weight and letting my muscles warm up. For the second I would settle down, pick up a little speed and take a moment (still walking) to admire the view. By the third quarter I was focused on speed and timings, and put all my effort into completing the course on time. Sometimes during the last quarter there would be time to slow down towards the end so that when the drill sergeant decided to send you off on another route immediately you could comply.

Hill Repetitions

Find a steep slope, which is at least 200 metres long

with an incline of around 30 degrees or more. It should take no more than a minute to sprint to the top. Sprint up the hill, then jog down to recover. Hill reps are designed to build your leg power and lung capacity. One hill rep is classified as 'sprint up, jog down'. Take short sharp steps and lean into the hill; relax as you jog down.

Press-ups

Press-ups could be called the mainstay of fitness – certainly as far as most armed services are concerned. Again, like all exercises, press-ups can be easy or hard but the important thing is to do them correctly.

➤   Lay face down, arms bent in the frog position, palms flat on the ground directly under the shoulders, body flush to the floor, legs and feet together.

➤   Raise your head, look forward and gently ease a rigid body off the floor using your arms. The position is correct when both the arms and body are straight.

➤   Relax in a controlled attitude by bending your arms back to the frog position.

The single most common mistake that is made by beginners is allowing the stomach and hips to sag. Although this will have the effect of making the exercise easier, it also removes 90 per cent of the benefit which defeats the whole object and makes the exercise pointless. Press-ups can be varied in a number of ways. For example, the feet can be raised on a step or low chair, or the hands can be placed closer together under the upper chest, both of which require a lot more effort.

You can do press-ups almost anywhere, all you need is a space that is as long as your body. Also, for such a simple exercise that requires no equipment, they work a whole range of body muscles from the neck down to the toes. If you are fairly new to exercise, start with just 10 press-ups and repeat as you feel able. When you feel fit enough increase the number to four bouts of 25 spread over your training session.

ALTERNATIVE EXERCISES

The basis of this book is to get fit while walking and running. However, from time to time there may be reasons why neither can done. It is therefore a good idea to have some form of back-up exercise, such as swimming and cycling. The frequency and duration of these exercises will depend on how long you cannot walk or run. If your programme has been interrupted due to an injury, see your doctor to check if you are fit enough to swim or cycle. Always make sure that any injury is fully healed before continuing a rigorous fitness programme.

Skipping

Skipping is a low risk, aerobic exercise that can be done by almost anyone, no matter what their weight or lack of fitness. It can be made as hard or easy as it needs to be. Athletes and performers of all kinds, from boxers to ballerinas, use skipping as part of their

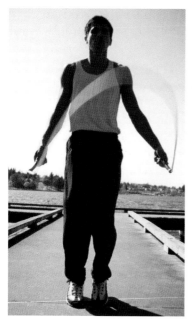

work-outs. This is because it provides hard exercise but without the risk of serious injury. Unlike jogging or running, skipping is regarded as a low-impact exercise.

The other advantage is that it only requires a skipping rope and a flat surface – no fancy equipment or expensive gym membership. The best type of rope to buy is a professional leather rope, which are inexpensive, are of the right weight and long-lasting. Even those who are as yet unable to jog or go on long walks due to breathing difficulty will still be able to participate gently in this exercise.

Start off slowly and aim to jump just high enough to clear the rope as it swings under your feet. Try and keep a constant rhythm without faltering for at least a minute then have a little rest. Once you have your breath back, skip again for another minute. Persistence will help to build up the lung capacity and muscles, and you will soon be able to skip for longer and longer. Once you are really proficient, try taking the knees higher as well.

Skip with both feet together or by taking running steps. Beginners tend to find it easier to run lightly on the balls of their feet, but once you get faster, jumping with both feet together on the spot will most probably be the preferred option. The rope itself should be swung by rotating the forearm and the wrist only, and making sure that the rope just skims the ground. At first many people leave the rope too slack, which then bounces on the floor and becomes tangled with the feet. Make sure that your elbows are tucked firmly into your waist and that you stand straight, with your shoulders back and your head up. Once you have reached the stage where you feel you have settled into a steady routine and speed, you should then attempt to do four sessions of between two and three minutes within an hour. This will not only greatly improve your lung capacity but it will also build up the muscles in your calves and lower legs – which will be a great benefit when you get on to the hillwalking.

Swimming

Apart from running over the hills every SAS soldier entering the Regiment must pass a basic swimming test. In the beginning this test is normally swimming fully clothed in the

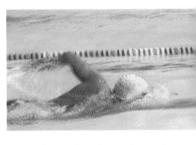

local baths, but later the annual test is often done by swimming a mile in the sea. For those who cannot swim there is usually a crash course. If you cannot swim, you are advised to go to your local swimming pool and enrol for a course. It is normally not expensive, and the students are put into groups according to age. The basics of swimming can be learnt in just a few lessons and improved at your leisure.

As with cycling there are several advantages of swimming. It is possible to swim while suffering from some form of injury as the water supports the body's weight. Swimming is also excellent for asthma sufferers as it does not provoke exercise-induced asthma.

Moreover, to get any real fitness benefit from swimming you need to swim relatively fast for at least half an hour at each session. While simply swimming up and down may feel good it will do little to improve your fitness. You should give yourself a time limit, for example, 30 minutes, and see how many lengths of the pool you can achieve in that time.

Cycling

Cycling is not part of SAS Selection, but is an excellent alternative to running. Indeed, you can cycle when suffering from leg strains caused by running. The distance covered on a bike is roughly five times that of running, although both are achieved with the equivalent energy burn.

Choose where you cycle with care. Cycling in traffic is dangerous and unpleasant, while mountain biking is very prone to accidents. A hard-surface route fairly free of traffic is ideal. You must always wear a cycling helmet. If you intend to do long distances on a racing bike, padded shorts are essential, as is a water-bottle. As with running, it is time in the saddle that is

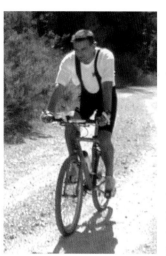

important. If you are not used to cycling, take it easy to start with, and make sure the bike is adjusted to suit your body and pedal stride. Begin with short (five-mile) routes and build up the distance slowly. This will give the muscle groups around the upper thigh and buttock time to become active. Get used to anticipating the inclines and declines ahead of you and so adjust your gearing.

FIVE-WEEK NORMAL FITNESS PROGRAMME

WEEK ONE

Monday–Friday
Morning:
3-mile walk;
skip for 3 min;
2 x 20 press-ups;
2 x 30 sit-ups

Evening:
Repeat morning
exercise

Saturday

Morning:　　　　　　　　*Evening:*
5-mile jog　　　　　　　Rest

Sunday

Morning:　　　　　　　Evening:
Rest　　　　　　　　　Rest

WEEK TWO/THREE

Monday

Morning:　　　　　　　　*Evening:*
5-mile jog　　　　　　　Swim 15 lengths

Tuesday

Morning:　　　　　　　　*Evening:*
5-mile jog　　　　　　　Skip for 10 min.

Wednesday

Morning:　　　　　　　　*Evening:*
3-mile best effort　　　　Skip for 10 min.

Thursday

Morning:　　　　　　　　*Evening:*
5-mile jog, best effort　　Swim 15 lengths

Friday

Morning:　　　　　　　　*Evening:*
20 hill reps of　　　　　Skip for 10 min.
200 metres

Saturday
Morning: *Evening:*
3-mile best effort   Rest

Sunday
Morning: *Evening:*
Rest   Rest

WEEK FOUR

Monday
Morning: *Evening:*
5-mile jog   Swim 15 lengths
(increase speed)

Tuesday
Morning: *Evening:*
Skip for 10 min;   Repeat morning
3 x 20 press-ups;   exercise
3 x 30 sit-ups

Wednesday
Morning: *Evening:*
Rest   Rest

Thursday
Morning: *Evening:*
5-mile jog, best effort   Skip for 10 min.

Friday
Morning:
5-mile jog

Evening:
Swim 15 lengths

Saturday
Morning:
Rest

Evening:
Rest

Sunday
Morning:
Rest

Evening:
Rest

AUTHOR'S NOTE

➤   I am now into my second month, having repeated the Weight-loss Programme while I was writing this chapter. I have lost almost two stone since I started, but am still a little overweight. I now feel ready to participate in regular physical exercise. The sit-up machine has proved a great bonus as it has firmed up my stomach muscles giving me a much slimmer profile. My next goal is to complete the Five-week Programme, finishing with a 15-mile mountain walk.

WEEK FIVE

Monday

Morning:	*Evening:*
6-mile jog & walk with rucksack Time: 1 hour 45 min.	Skip for 10 min.; 3 x 20 press-ups; 3 x 30 sit-ups

Tuesday

Morning:	*Evening:*
Rest	Rest

Wednesday

Morning:	*Evening:*
8-mile jog & walk with rucksack Time: 2 hours 15 min.	Rest

Thursday

Morning:	*Evening:*
5-mile jog, best effort	5-mile comfortable jog

Friday

Morning:	*Evening:*
Rest	Swim 15 lengths

Saturday

Morning:	*Evening:*
10-mile jog & walk with rucksack Time: 3 hours 30 min.	Rest

Sunday

Morning:
15-mile jog & walk
with rucksack
Time: 3 hours 30 min.

Evening:
Rest

MUSCLE STRENGTH AND STAMINA

In addition to cardio-respiratory fitness, those soldiers attempting SAS Selection require a high level of muscular strength and endurance, as many SAS operations require the carrying of heavy loads (e.g. rucksacks) over great distances. Muscular strength is the greatest amount of force a muscle or muscle group can exert in a single effort. Muscular endurance is the ability of a muscle or muscle group to do repeated contractions against a less-than-maximum resistance for a given time. Although muscular endurance and strength are separate fitness components, they are closely related. Progressively working against resistance will produce gains in both of these components. This can be achieved by:

➤ Isometric contractions which produces contraction but no movement, as whenpushing against an immovable object. Force is produced with no change in the angle of the joint.

➤ Isotonic contractions which causes a joint to move through a range of motion against a constant resistance. Examples of this are push-ups, sit-ups, and the lifting of weights.

27479

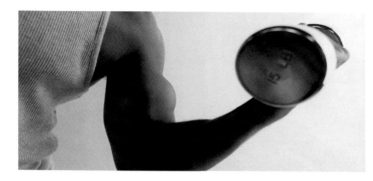

For a muscle to increase in strength the workload to which it is subjected during exercise must be increased beyond what is normally encountered – this is known as muscle overload. Muscles acclimatize to increased workloads by becoming larger and stronger and by developing greater endurance. This is accomplished by using an exercise weight which lets you do 8 to 12 repetitions of a particular exercise correctly before the muscle becomes fatigued. Finding the correct weight for each exercise is a matter of trial and error and will vary from individual to individual. In principle if you cannot carry out three repetitions of a particular exercise, the weight is too heavy and should be reduced. If you are able to carry out 20 repetitions without muscle fatigue, then the weight is too light. Initially, you should choose a weight resistance that lets you do no more than 12 repetitions of a given exercise.

A sustained training program using the correct weight will significantly improve muscle endurance and strength. The key to overloading a muscle is to make that muscle work harder than it normally does. When an overload is applied to a muscle, it adapts by becoming stronger and/or by improving its endurance. An overload may be achieved by any of the following methods:

➤ Increasing the weight.
➤ Increasing the number of repetitions.
➤ Increasing the number of sets.
➤ Decreasing the rest time between sets.
➤ Speed of exercise movement.

As with all forms of exercise results depend on the individual, but in principle muscle fitness can only be achieved by progressively increasing the weight, number of repetitions and number of repetition sets. When you can correctly do the upper limit of repetitions for the set without reaching muscle failure, it is time to increase the resistance. For most people this upper limit should be 12 repetitions.

ADDING WEIGHT

➤ If the exercise calls for 12 repetitions, once this can be achieved correctly without muscle fatigue, the weight should be increased by around 10%. As the weight and number of repetition sets increase, reduce the additional weight to 5%.

Muscular fitness is not something that can be done on an ad-hoc basis because sporadic exercise may do more harm than good. You can only maintain a level of muscular fitness by doing the appropriate workouts at least three times a week. In addition you should continue to exercise the same muscle groups with each session, when different muscle groups are exercised at each workout, the principle of regularity is violated and gains in strength are negligible.

If you intend to carry out muscular fitness training on a daily basis then you should make sure that each daily session involves exercising different muscle groups. It is important that you allow the individual muscle groups time to recover, as continued resistance training for the same muscle group can be harmful. There should be at least a 48-hour recovery period between workouts for the same muscle groups. Likewise during the session, you should also rest between different sets of exercises. This rest period will depend on the intensity of the workout, in the early stages 30 seconds should be enough but as you progress increase your rest between

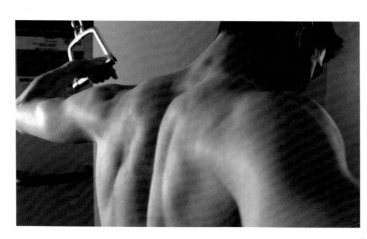

individual sets by up to 2 minutes

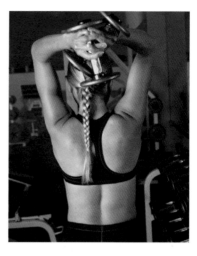

Muscles work and contract in different ways, some push while others pull or rotate. Whatever their function your training programme should be designed to work all the major muscle groups. Many muscles are organized into opposing pairs; activating one muscle results in a pulling motion, while activating the opposing muscle results in the opposite, or pushing, movement. Where possible organize your exercise sets so that a pushing or lifting motion (overhead press) is balanced constriction during the down side of the exercise. The best sequence to follow for a total-body strength workout is to first exercise the muscles of the hips and legs, followed by the muscles of the upper back and chest, then the arms, abdominal, low back, and neck. As long as all muscle groups are exercised at the proper intensity, improvement will occur. Using an even-handed set of exercises will help balance the muscle build and reduce the risk of injury.

SAFETY

Muscular fitness training can cause injury either through using an excessive weight or by doing the exercise incorrectly. Where possible you should always carry out this kind of training when there are others around to observe your progress, better still exercise with a partner, and in this way any improper techniques or potential danger should be spotted. A common problem when training in a gym is to try and lift weights far in excess of your capacity. For those just beginning a programme this can be disheartening, so always start by using the correct weight for you, not what others can lift. Breathing should be constant during exercise, exhale as you lift or pull the muscle and inhale as you relax.

As with all forms of fitness training, maintaining a level of enthusiasm and interest play a major factor. Motivation and determination may well be the prime factors in this but planning a varied programme will

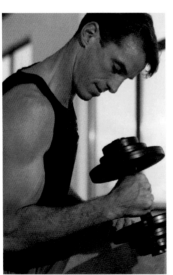

help to maintain your resolve and prevent the training becoming to boring. Using different equipment, changing the exercises and altering the volume and intensity are good ways to add variety, which in the long term may also produce better results

Muscle exercises can be done in three basic ways; resistance apparatus (multi-exercise station), individual weights, and partner-resisted exercises. Ideally, you should choose one method of muscle-resistance training and stick to it for the duration of your programme. If you are able to visit a gym then you will have the choice of all three, although more than likely you will choose either a multi-exercise station or weights. However, where you are not able to visit a gym and the equipment is not available (financial considerations do not allow) you may be able to carry out a resistance training programme using a partner. Interchanging between methods is not a good idea as there is a difference in the type of muscle overload experienced, which could have an adverse affect

WHAT EXERCISES?

The method of training you choose will determine the range of exercises open to you. In all cases you should start with about eight basic exercises which should exercise the muscles of the arms, shoulders, middle body and legs. Choose those exercises which work on several different muscle groups at the same time as opposed to individual muscle groups. These are determined by the number of joints involved in the repetition – multi-joint repetitions work more muscle groups

TRAINING PERIOD

For those people new to resistance training, the programme should be broken down into sections. These sections are categorized into three levels:

foundation, conditioning and maintenance. Foundation level is at the start of your programme and lasts for about one week. At this level you should concentrate on doing each exercise in the correct way, and this is best achieved by using a lighter resistance. This will ensure you get used to the exercise movement without causing undue strain or injury. A maximum of three workouts with a reduced number of repetitions (6–8) for each exercise is best. During the second week the number of workouts should be increased to five while extending the repetitions (8–12). If you can complete 12 repetitions without strain then the resistance/weight should be increased slightly. During the foundation level you should aim to complete just one set of each exercise using a comfortable resistance/weight, concentrating mainly on the ease of movement

Conditioning starts in the third week. This is where the real work is done. The resistance/weight should be increased to the point where 12 repetitions are just possible. Once the muscle has become acclimatized, i.e. you are able to do more than 12 repetitions without strain, you should increase the number of sets to two with a 30-second recovery time between each set. As you progress through week four you should aim to increase the number of sets to three. Once this has been accomplished it is time to start adding additional resistance/weight. As previously mentioned the weight increase at this stage should not exceed five per cent. By the end of week six you should see a significant increase in the amount of muscle strength and endurance. However, for general fitness three repetitions of each exercise is considered to be enough, keep in mind that muscle fitness needs to be maintained.

Maintenance of muscular fitness requires the ongoing commitment of resistance/weigh training. Once you have reached the desired level of fitness you should adjust your workouts accordingly. Most muscle groups once trained can be held at their present level by two workouts a week as the emphasis is no longer on progression but on retention. Once your ideal level has been realized consider combining aerobic exercise to your weekly fitness schedule, this will greatly enhance the whole body

DEFINITIONS

➤ Resistance/weight is related directly to the amount of muscle contractions required to move that resistance/weight a given distance, usually the maximum length or movement of the functioning body joint.

➤ Repetitions refer to the action of the body or parts of the body during a single muscular exercise. The number of repetitions and resistance/weight define when muscle overload is reached.

➤ A set consists of a given number of repetitions (normally 8 -12) in any given exercise. A set can be freely completed (no time limit) or timed i.e. 12 curls in 20 seconds. The same exercise set can be repeated several times with a rest period in between.

(contd)

➤ A given number of sets in different exercises are called a workout. A number of workouts per week over a period of several weeks is a programme. The following section is an example of a resistance/weight training using the body's major muscle groups.

POINTS ON RESISTANCE TRAINING

➤ Workout with a friend or with a group.

➤ Schedule time for your workout.

➤ Breathe when lifting. Exhale during the concentric (positive) phase of contraction, and inhale during the eccentric (negative) phase.

➤ Do all exercises in a controlled manner.

➤ Accuracy is better than speed.

➤ Exercise several muscle groups at the same time where possible.

➤ Increase the number of sets before increasing resistance/weights.

➤ Rest from 30 to 180 seconds between different sets.

➤ Allow at least 48 hours of recovery between workouts

➤ Never increase the resistance/weight by more than 10% at a time.

➤ Use alternate pulling and pushing exercises.

TRAINING WITHOUT SPECIAL EQUIPMENT

All forms of lifting, pushing, turning and carrying

provide resistance to the muscles. What causes the resistance is of little concern to the muscle groups; however they work harder, they adapt. But there is a distinct difference between hard manual work and exercising in a gym in as much that the latter has an organized programme aimed at balanced muscle development. It is possible to use a partner in muscle-resistance exercises, performing exercises where their weight is the opposing resistance. The more a pair of partners workout together, the more effective they become in providing the proper resistance for each exercise. The resister must apply enough resistance to bring the exerciser to muscle failure in 8 to 12 repetitions.

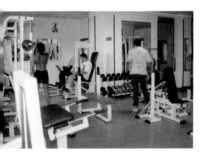

By far the best way to achieve increased muscular strength and endurance is to use a gym. Even the most basic gymnasiums have a weight room with equipment for resistance-training exercises, while the more up-to-date establishments supply specialist resistance-training machines. If you are new to the equipment, you should seek advice to ensure the correct weight and techniques are used for each exercise.

As resistance training is an ongoing activity you may consider purchasing your own equipment. Most large supermarkets now supply a complete range of good equipment from the simple bar-bells to a complete fitness station. Providing you have the room at home you should consider the cost as many gymnasiums can be expensive to join. If you do go down this road remember to have someone act as spotter in the event of injury.

GYM vs HOME EQUIPMENT

There is some debate about where you should exercise, in a gym or in your own home. The gym offers you an environment where you can learn from others, which is especially valuable if you are new to exercise or have no exercise partner. On the other hand there is the cost both in time and money. Enrolment is usually for a minimum of six months and few people have a gym on their doorstep. However, a gym will have a greater range of equipment as well as professional staff to provide advice and, in most cases, to monitor your progress.

There are people who wish to become fit and for a variety of personal reasons do not want to expose themselves in a gym. This can be a very real dilemma as many individuals can find some physical defect in themselves that they do not wish to share with strangers.

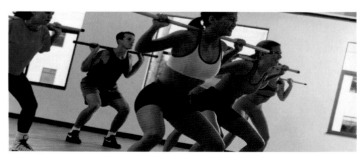

Common among these are:

➤ Obesity.

➤ Age.

➤ Poor body stature.

➤ Sex

Walking into a gym as a beginner can be an unnerving experience. Your first glance takes in the fanatics who are working out like some demented robot, then the slim and very attractive young women who cast you a sympathetic look. However, you should not let this put you off, most gyms offer an excellent service, with staff that would sooner help you than talk to the posers.

If you feel you are not yet ready to face the gym, then you could consider working out at home. While this saves time and allows you to exercise at differing periods throughout the day, it also requires a lot more discipline.

Most people go off and buy several items of equipment after seeing them advertised and are convinced that several minutes a day will provide them with the body they desire. In reality the equipment usually ends up gathering dust in the garage or spare room. If you intend to exercise at home, make sure you think it through and know exactly what it is you hope to achieve before buying any equipment

Treadmills

Treadmills are basically a moving belt on which you

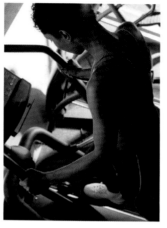

walk. Again these come in a variety of shapes and sizes some are powered by an electric motor and some have a mechanical action. In honesty the only reason for having a treadmill in your home is for use during bad weather, apart from that you will reap far more benefit from walking or running through the park which is free.

Bikes

The exercise bike is very similar to the treadmill except it has one main advantage in as much that it is beneficial to use in the home. The cost of purchasing a normal bike is about the same, but there is the added risk of having an accident while riding in the traffic. Either way, both static exercise bikes and road bikes will prove of great benefit to your training programme. If you intend to exercise indoors place the bike so that it faces the television, this will help remove the monotony so that you endure a longer exercise period.

Free Weights

These are the original exercise equipment and until the advent of exercise resistance machines very much the backbone of the fitness industry. They come in two basic forms bar-bells (individual hand weights)

134

and free weights (a bar with equal weights either end) both are simple and fairly cheap to purchase. These are still good for building muscle strength and endurance

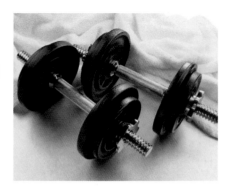

Multi Exercise Station

In recent years there has been a growth in the use of multi-exercise stations or variable resistance weight machines, many of which are now available in most good gymnasiums. These are pieces of equipment designed to do a number of different exercises. At the top end of the scale a good quality multi-exercise station will put the whole body through a series of exercises designed to work all the muscle groups. The added advantage of these machines is their ability to vary the resistance of each exercise, putting the muscle under tolerable but not excessive tension during the tension and relaxation phase of each exercise. Another big advantage of a multi-exercise

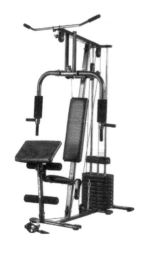

station is its safety over the more traditional free weights which you could become trapped under or suffer an injury if one falls on you. Weight machines are extremely safe as the bulk of exercises are controlled via a pulley system that has a preset stop position which allows individuals to train at home or unsupervised. A further benefit of working out on a weight machine is that most of your routine can be done in the same place. Additionally, such machines can be adjusted to compensate for the beginner through to the fittest person by moving a pin to vary the resistance.

Where time is a factor in achieving a good fitness programme it may be worthwhile considering the purchase of weights or a weight machine for use at home. When compared to the cost of enrolling in a fitness club for a year, they can be very cost effective, added to which you can exercise when convenient and save time travelling to your gym. Most larger supermarkets now carry a good range of fitness and exercise equipment at a variety of prices depending on the model and its complexity.

Whether you choose to exercise in the home or in a gym you should seek advice and exercise with caution and supervision until you become proficient

EXERCISE CHART

The following examples will help you select the most suitable exercises for developing good muscular endurance and strength. The exercises described here include free weights, weight machines and supporting equipment.

Dumb-bell Raise

Grip a 5kg (11lb) dumb-bell in each hand and stand upright with your feet slightly apart. Hold the weights at your thighs; knuckles outward. Raise each dumb-bell in turn lifting in an arch from your thigh to your ear. Hold the position for about 2 seconds then lower and repeat with the other arm (10 repetitions each arm) Do not let the body go into a rocking motion.

Dumb-bell Press

Grip a 5kg (11lb) dumb-bell in each hand and stand upright with your feet slightly apart. Curl in your arms until you are holding the weights bay your ears: knuckles out. Raise each dumb-bell in turn above your head, pushing it over towards the opposite shoulder, hold for 2 seconds then lower and repeat with the other arm (10 repetitions each arm).

Dumb-bell Side Swing

Grip a 5 kg (11lb) dumb-bell in each hand and sit on a firm bench. Recline so that your back is flat on the bench with your feet firmly on the ground, slightly apart. Raise the weights above your shoulders keeping the arms straight. From this position lower the weights by moving your arms out to the

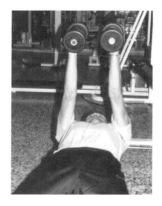

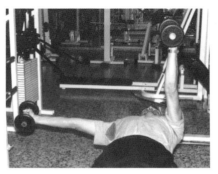

side. Hold the position for 2 seconds at maximum strain before returning to the above shoulder position, (10 repetitions). Make sure the arms are lowered parallel to the shoulders do not let then drift towards the stomach or over the head.

Dumb-bell Over-head Swing

Grip a 7kg (15lb) dumb-bell and sit on a firm bench. Recline so that your back is flat on the bench and your legs are positioned either side for balance. Hold the dumb-bell with both hands raising it with straight arms above your shoulders. From this position lower your arms over your head to maximum stretch and hold this position for 2 seconds before returning to the above shoulder position (10 repetitions).

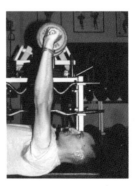
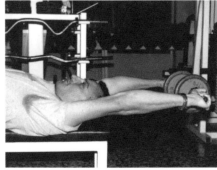

Dumb-bell Under-Arm Curl

Grip a 7kg (15lb) dumb-bell in your right hand and bend forward, feet slightly apart, placing your left hand on a bench for support. Let the weight hang straight down without dropping the shoulder. Curl the wrist inwards raising the dumbbell under the armpit. Hold and maximum strain for 2 seconds then return to the arm stretched position (10 repetitions each arm). Change arms and repeat. Don't let the shoulders dip.

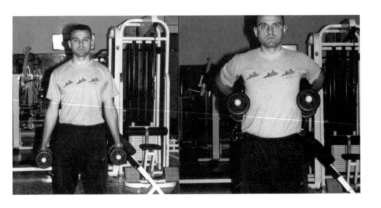

Bent Leg Dead-lift

Select a 30-40 kg (66-88lb) total weight. Stand with the weights level in front of your toes, feet slightly apart. Bend the knees keeping your back straight and grip the bar (overhand). Lift he weight by straightening the knees, keeping the back arched while pushing the shoulders back. Once in the upright position hold the weight at waist height for 2 seconds then lower under the same control as you lifted (10 repetitions). Equal care should be taken when lowering the weights as lifting them.

Front Arm Curls

Select a 10kg (22lb) total weight. Stand with the weights level in front of your toes, feet slightly apart. Bend the knees keeping your back straight and grip the bar (underhand). Lift he weight by straightening the knees, keeping the back arched while pushing the shoulders back, until it is at waist height. From this position raise the bar until it is shoulder height, hold for 2 seconds and return to the waist (10 repetitions).

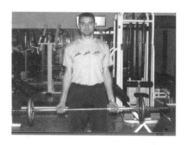 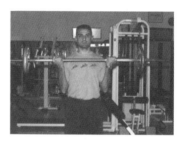

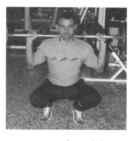

Squat

Select a 30 - 40 kg (66-88lb) weight. Stand with your feet apart, grip the bar overhand, then bending the knees and keeping your back straight, lift the weight over your head to rest on your shoulders. Bend your knees until the thighs are parallel to the ground; keep the head and shoulders upright and your back straight. Hold for 2 seconds and then straighten. Do 8 to 12 repetitions or until muscle failure. Place a flat 5cm block under the heels for improved steadiness.

Bench Press

Select a 35 - 45 kg (77-99lb) weight and place in the stands at the end of a bench. Recline so that your back is flat on the bench and your legs are positioned either side for balance. Lift the bar with (overhand grip) with your hands slightly wider than should width. Hold the bar directly above your chest arms fully extended. Slowly lower the bar to your chest, hold for 2 seconds and raise. Do 8 to 12 repetitions or until muscle failure. Make sure this exercised is assisted, supervised or watched by another person.

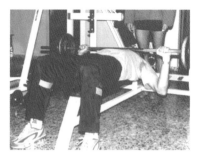
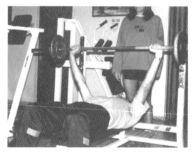

Bent-over Row

Select a 30 - 40 kg (66-88lb) weight. Bend forward keeping your back straight letting your arms hand down from the shoulders. Flex the knees so that you are able to grip the bar (overhand) in comfortable manner. Bend the elbows lifting the weight into the waist and hold for 2 seconds before returning to the starting position. Do 8 to 12 repetitions or until muscle failure.

Wrist Curls

Place a 10 -15 kg (22-33lb) weight on a small bench. Kneel in front of the bench so that you can grip the weight (underhand) with your wrist and forearms resting on the bench. Keeping the elbows stationary, curl the fingers and then the wrist to maximum strain, hold and then relax. Do 8 to 12 repetitions or until muscle failure.

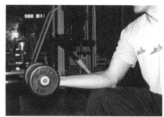

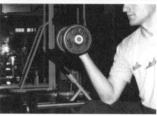

Leg Press (multi exercise station)

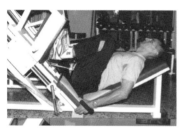

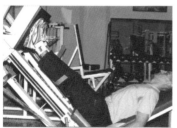

Sit at the leg press potion after selecting a 30kg (66lb) resistance weight. Your legs should not be bent more than 90 degrees with the balls of your feet flat against the resister. Push the weight until your legs are straight but without locking the knees. Return to the starting position in a controlled manner. Do 8 to 12 repetitions or until muscle failure.

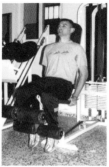 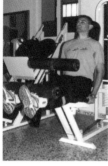

Leg Extension (multi exercise station)

After selecting a 30kg (66lb) resistance weight, sit in the position with your lower legs behind the padded resister. Hold onto the handles if provided or grip the seat, making sure you keep your body in the upright position. Straighten your legs to maximum strain, hold and then return to the start position.

Leg Curl (multi exercise station)

Adjust the resistance weight to 15kg (33lb) Lie on your stomach with your legs extended down the bench under the padded resister. Maintain body position by gripping the handles provided or the sides of the bench. Flex your legs at the knee bringing the heels as close to the buttocks as possible, then return to the starting position. Do 8 to 12 repetitions or until muscle failure.

Bench Press (multi exercise station)

Adjust the weight to 35 - 45 kg (77-99lb). Recline so that your back is flat on the bench and your legs are positioned either side for balance. The lifting bar should be located at the lower half of the chest. Grip the bar (underhand).

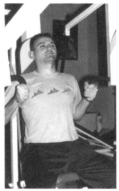 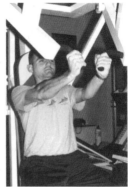

Lift the bar until your arms are fully extended. Slowly lower the bar to your chest. Do 8 to 12 repetitions or until muscle failure.

Biceps Curl (multi exercise station)

Adjust the resistance weight to 25kg (55lb). Regulate the bar so that there is no resistance when you hold it (palms out) at groin height. Your body should be straight, arms extended and feet slightly apart.
Exercise: Bend your forearms only without moving the elbows bringing the bar to chest level, then lower under control to the start position. Do 8 to 12 repetitions or until muscle failure.

Seated Row (multi exercise station)

Adjust the resistance weight to 25kg (55lb). Sit with your feet firmly against the apparatus gripping (overhand) the resister bar. Keep your back straight with your knees slightly bent.
Exercise: Pull the bar back to the lower chest while flexing the elbows outwards at chest height. Return to the start position under control. Do 8 to 12 repetitions or until muscle failure. Keep the body immobile using only the arms for this exercise.

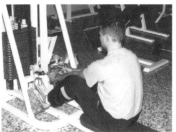
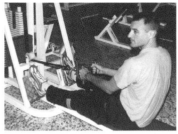

Lat Pull Down (multi exercise station)

Adjust the weight to 25kg (55lb). You can stand, sit or kneel for this exercise depending on the apparatus. Grip the bar above your head so that the palms are away from the body.

Exercise: Pull the bar down until it rests on the back of your shoulders, then return to the start position under control. Do 8 to 12 repetitions or until muscle failure.

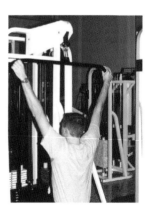
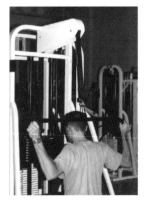

Incline Sit-up (multi exercise station)

Set the bench to the required incline and position yourself with your knees bent at a 90-degree angle to your feet which should be anchored with a strap. Interlace you fingers behind your head. Flex your torso and curl forwards as far a possible, then return to the starting position. Do 25 to 50 repetitions or until muscle failure. If you can do 50 sit-ups without strain, increase the incline on the bench to the next rung.

Chin up

Adjust the beam until it is at least 15cm above your outstretched height. Jump up and grip the beam so that you are in the hanging position. Where a high beam is not available bend your knees to clear the floor. Using your arms pull your body up until your chin has cleared the beam. Return to the hanging position under control. Do 12 to 15 repetitions or until muscle failure. If you can do more than 20 repetitions without muscle strain try placing a weighted belt around your waist.

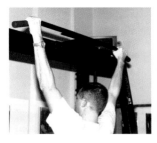

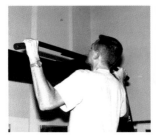

WEIGHT TRAINING PROGRAMMES

There are three stages in weight training: beginner, intermediate and advanced. The approach is fairly standard, starting with a weight you can handle, then increasing the amount of repetitions and the weight. Always work with a weight that is comfortable, and remember to warm-up before starting (see Flexibility, p.97). The examples shown here are only a guide; try to make your own programme working as many muscle groups as possible.

BEGINNER

Exercise	Repetitions	Sets
Dumb-bell raise.	8	3
Dumb-bell side swing.	8	3
Squat	5	3
Bench press	5	3
Bent over row	5	3
Seated row	8	3
Incline sit-up	5	3
Chin-up	5	3

INTERMEDIATE

Exercise	Repetitions	Sets
Dumb-bell raise.	10	3
Dumb-bell press	10	3
Dumb-bell side swing.	10	3
Squat.	8	3
Bent leg dead lift.	5	3
Bench press.	8	3
Bent over row.	8	3

Seated row.	10	3
Leg press	10	3
Leg extension	10	3
Incline sit-up	8	3
Lat pull-down.	10	3
Chin-up.	8	3

ADVANCED

Exercise	Repetitions	Sets
Dumb-bell raise.	12	3
Dumb-bell overhead swing.	12	3
Dumb-bell press.	12	3
Dumb-bell side swing.	12	3
Dumb-bell underarm curls	10	3
Squat	10	3
Bent leg dead lift	10	3
Front arm curls	10	3
Wrist curls	12	3
Bench press	10	3
Bent over row	10	3
Seated row	12	3
Leg press.	12	3
Leg extension.	12	3
Incline sit-up	12	3
Lat pull down	12	3
Leg curls	12	3
Chin-up	10	3

Programme Two

Soldiers who wish to join the SAS must first spend a weekend at Hereford where they are briefed on the qualities required by the SAS. This briefing takes place some six months prior to the soldier actually attending Selection and gives them time to achieve the required fitness level. The following chapter is loosely based on the fitness schedule issued on the Special Forces Briefing Course (SFBC). Those who have completed Programme One of this book should now be ready to tackle some serious training.

Unlike the earlier programmes where the maximum effort was a fast jog, now you have to run. Run fast, run uphill, run downhill, run in the rain, snow and sun and run with a bergen. It sounds arduous and that's because it is. However, taking into account that we are not actually joining the SAS, we can modify the programme to make it much more enjoyable.

Vary the length of the routes to take into account your age and physical condition, and once you have reached a standard of fitness, push yourself a little bit further. Walk up hills and jog down them, don't run; it is always a good idea to keep a little bit of energy in reserve. Once a week, perhaps on a Sunday morning, try doubling you distance. We can do this by choosing our own routes and setting our own times and goals. But these goals must be met.

PREPARATION

There are no special SAS secrets to passing Selection: there is only the reality. For all the soldiers this reality comes down to age and how well they have prepared themselves. Their chances of success are greater if they are under thirty years of age. Likewise those that have spent their days in a sedentary occupation, sitting behind desk for example, have little chance of succeeding

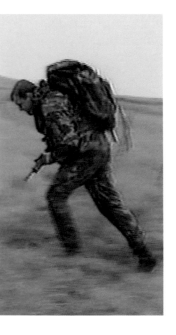

because there are no short cuts. There is a great deal of truth in the saying: 'No pain, no gain.' The SAS has seen many candidates arrive at Hereford thinking that they have found 'magic formulas' and short cuts to make them better performers. These hypochondriacs bring with them all sorts of vitamin pills, supplements and concoctions, believing them to be superior to a good training routine and diet – they all fail.

Before you take to the hills with your rucksack make sure you are prepared. Apart from your fitness and diet preparations you will need to learn several other skills, such as how to read a map and use a compass accurately enabling you to navigate well. This skill is particularly useful when the visibility is poor; and talking of visibility, an understanding of weather will also be helpful when you trekking across the hills.

NEW TO HILLWALKING

In the normal course of events, hillwalking is not dangerous; on the contrary in many ways it is far safer than the cities. It is the isolation factor that presents the greatest threat, but so long as a few simple rules are obeyed you should have no problem. If you opt for a pre-planned route, such as from a guide book, then any problems will be indicated and the appropriate action obvious. If you have chosen your own route, you should make sure you don't put yourself too far from safety.

HILLWALKING SAFETY

➤ Never travel alone.

➤ Always tell someone sensible where you are going and your estimated time of return.

➤ Always have a contingency plan for bad weather.

➤ Carry a first-aid kit.

➤ Carry a mobile phone if you have one.

➤ Do not take unnecessary risks.

➤ Learn to read a map and use a compass.

➤ Dress and carry the appropriate clothing and equipment.

GOOD NAVIGATION

It is important to master both map reading and navigation skills if you intend to participate in cross-country exercises similar to that endured on SAS Selection. Not only will such skills reduce your chances of getting lost, they will also enable you to find the shortest way and the best terrain to get from one point to another.

Navigation can be done in two basic ways. The best known and the most traditional is to use a map and a compass. A more modern method is to use a Global Positioning System. Although the latter may seem more appealing, it can be costly and if the batteries run down at an inopportune moment, you could be in trouble. Therefore, though both methods are covered here, more emphasis will be put on the proper use of a map and compass. This is an important skill and should be learnt by anyone taking part in any outdoor fitness pursuit.

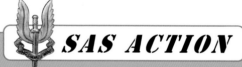

SAS ACTION

➤ While fitness is the main requirement topass into the ranks of the
SAS, good navigation comes a close
second. It is essential that map
information be fully recognized and
its representation in relation to
your route be understood.

Ordnance Survey maps

Without a good map it is
easy to get lost in the
countryside. For
example, a right of
way may become
obscured by
undergrowth
and crops, but a
map will be able
to show you
where it should be.
Of all the maps available the
best are Ordnance Survey (OS)
maps, because these are often more
detailed than those found in guide books
and the like. Ordnance Survey maps come in
different scales; most commonly 1:50,000. While
these are good in their own right and show the public
rights of way (marked in red), the best scale to use for
cross-country walking is the 1:25,000 Pathfinder map.
This larger scale not only shows the rights of way
(marked in green), but will also show other useful
details such as way-marked routes, camp sites,
permissable paths and some areas of open access.

Ordnance Survey maps also show roads, tracks and
paths other than those defined as public rights of way.
Just because they are shown on the map does not
necessarily mean that the public are free to use them.
This is clearly stated on the map itself: 'the
representation on this map of any other road, track
or path is no evidence of the existence of a right of

way.' However, in general practice these routes are often travelled along without any hindrance. If the landowners really don't want you there, they will usually put up signs to that effect.

You may notice that some of the lanes and tracks on the map are uncoloured. These 'white roads', as they are sometimes called, often lead to a remote farmhouse or country mansion and as such are normally private. Careful study of the map should give you the answers, but if you are unsure, ask the local authority for advice.

Most maps will give an idea of the 'relief' of an area by showing various heights as contour lines. These are shown as continuous brown lines, with each line defining a certain height (this height will be shown at some point along the line). By studying the contour lines, you will see that as well as showing the height, they also give an idea of the shape of any hill or mountain. If you wish to stay on the level rather than negotiating sharp inclines and declines, use the contours on your map to plan your route. Following a contour where possible is often easier than following a straight line.

Map Symbols

Map symbols represent objects or places on the ground, for example, a telephone box is marked on the map with capital 'T', while a church with a spire will be represented by a black dot with a cross on top. Rivers and streams are marked in blue with their thickness giving some indication as to size. The routes in this book are normally indicated with a three- or four-figure grid reference which are qualified by the object on the ground. However, not all objects are visibly represented, for example, a trig-point is a man-made fixed concrete object normally on the top of a hill or mountain, while a spot-height only indicates the height of a particular hill above sea level.

Compass

Compasses all work on the principle of having a magnetized needle constantly pointing to North. There are many varieties on the market varying in size and price, but the one most useful for outdoor navigation is the 'Silva'-type compass. This is generally made from clear plastic and is rectangular in shape. The actual compass part is off-set to the left-hand side, while the base contains a magnifying glass and various scales to calculate grid references. The rim of the compass housing can be rotated and is marked with degrees or mil or sometimes both.

As compasses work on the principle of magnetic attraction to the North Pole, it also means that any localized magnetic source will have an effect on your needle; this includes electricity cables, pylons or any heavy metal object. To prevent such sensitivity, some manufacturers fill the compass housing with

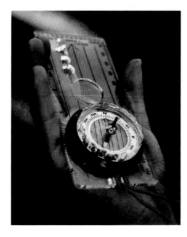

fluid. These often contain a bubble, but as long as it isn't too large, it will not affect the working of the compass.

Setting a Map by Inspection

First find a landmark that is both obvious and not likely to disappear overnight; a mountain, river or a road would do the job. Then take a look at your map and find your chosen feature. Once it has been located, simply align the map to the landmark and you will see the other features around you fall into place.

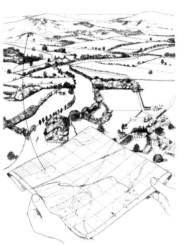

Setting A Map by Compass

Lay one of the flat edges of your compass along a North-South grid line on your map. Keeping hold of both the map and the compass, turn both until the needle of the compass is pointing North. Check the surrounding landmarks around you: they should now conform to those on the map.

Finding a Grid Reference

All maps have grid lines, which are vertical and horizontal thin blue lines superimposed over the terrain. The vertical lines are called 'eastings' because they are numbered from west to east. The horizontal lines are called 'northings' because they are numbered from south to north. These lines intersect and create squares of a defined area. For example, on a 1:50,000 Landranger map the areas defined by the grid lines are 1 km square.

A grid reference will pinpoint a precise area on the map using both the easting and the northing numbers. The reference of a grid square will consist of four numbers: the first two will be the number shown on the left-hand grid line – the easting – and the second two numbers will be those shown in the middle of the bottom line – the northing. As an example, the grid square in the illustration is 1562. Map references are always given with the easting number first followed by the northing. To find a point within the actual grid square, the square itself is divided up into tenths, so that half way across would be '5'. This number is then added after the relevant easting or northing reference so that an exact point can be located. To work out the tenths precisely, use the romer on your compass, or a protractor. An example of a six-figure grid reference is illustrated (right): the location shown can be read as GR155628.

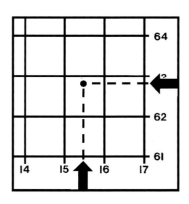

Taking a Compass Bearing from the Map

A bearing can be defined as the number of degrees in an angle measured clockwise from a fixed northern grid line. Compasses may be marked with 360 degrees, or, more usually, with 6400 mils. Bearings are used to keep you going in the right direction and are especially useful when visibility is bad.

To work out your route, take a good look at the map, noting the terrain, any potential obstacles such as bogs and the distance you will need to travel. Using obvious landmarks, such as a road or a bridge, divide your journey up into easily manageable sections. The point at which you are now, your start-point, should be labelled as 'A' and the landmark at the end of your first section should be labelled point 'B'. To take a bearing from A to B, draw a line between them and place one edge of your compass along it. Be sure that the direction of travel arrow is pointing in the

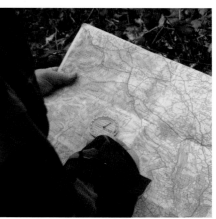

direction you want to go. With the base of the compass held securely in place, rotate the compass dial so that the engraved lines on the dial base lie parallel with the North–South grid lines on the map. Look once more

AUTHOR'S NOTE

➤ Contouring in fog or bad visibility can produce an interesting effect: most people tend to start wandering downhill. To counter this, make sure you take a few steps in an uphill direction every hundred metres or so. Remember that poor visibility will also mean that you move more slowly.

at the direction of travel arrow on the compass housing and read off the bearing next to it. All you will then need to do to use this bearing is to keep the magnetic arrow pointing North over the engraved arrow in the base. You will then be able to follow the direction of travel arrow to point B.

Keeping on Course

The direction of your route will depend upon certain factors: the type of terrain has already been mentioned, but the weather and the time of day will also need to be taken into consideration. If you know you will have good weather with good visibility, choose prominent landmarks that can be easily seen both by the naked eye and on the map. Once you have taken your bearing, in the way described above, find an obvious feature in line with the direction you're travelling in and head towards it. With this always in sight, you will not need to check your compass often to make sure that you are keeping on the right route. It will also help you to stay on track if you have to make a slight detour due to some unexpected obstacle. Although a compass is a useful tool, it should not rule you. Always try and keep a mental image of the terrain in your mind, as remembered from the map. With careful route planning and checking landmarks against the map every time you come to one, you should be confident that you will reach your final goal, whatever the weather.

Magnetic Variation

There are actually three 'Norths' known to science. True North is the fixed location of the North Pole, but this is rarely used for navigational purposes. Grid North is the North depicted on maps by the grid lines. However, Magnetic North is the one most commonly used by those engaged in outdoor pursuits. It is the alignment of the Earth's magnetic field that causes the needle in a compass always to point to Magnetic North. However, every year there are slight changes to the magnetic field and this will also cause the position of Magnetic North to vary. To

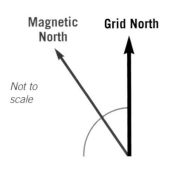

In 1998, Magnetic North was 4.5 degrees west of Grid North and this margin decreases by about 1 degree in 6 years

counteract this, you can use information shown on your map, such as the date it was printed and the degree of variation, to calculate the difference. The result must then be either added to or subtracted from Grid North to obtain an accurate bearing.

MAGNETIC VARIATION

The way to remember variation is:

➤ Mag to Grid = Get Rid
Subtract the variation from your compass bearing before applying it to the map.

➤ Grid to Mag = Add
Add the variation to your map bearing before applying it to your compass.

Although some people insist that calculating this degree of variation is essential, for most normal purposes, such as hillwalking, it is hardly necessary. In fact, over a small distance the difference is just about negligible anyway. The best solution to this problem is to shorten the sections of your route, so ensuring that your bearings still retain a good degree of accuracy. On the other hand, if you insist on working out the magnetic variation, bear in mind that it will take you extra time and there is a high risk that you could make an error which will throw you completely off course. Personally, I have never bothered to work out the magnetic variation unless I have been attempting a long trek over barren, featureless countryside.

Putting a Compass Bearing on the Map

Sometimes even the best navigators lose their bearings. But there is something you can do to relocate your position on a map by using a compass and a couple of landmarks. First of all pick out two easily identifiable features and pinpoint them on your map. Next, take your compass and point it at the first landmark. Hold it firmly and turn the housing until the orientating arrow is aligned with the magnetic needle. Now you should be able to read off the bearing to the landmark.

To take an example, the bearing to the first landmark is 5700 mils. If we calculate the magnetic variation, which, for this example, we'll say is 40 mils, this needs to be subtracted from the bearing, leaving a revised figure of 5660 mils. Adjust the compass dial to this amount. On the map, place the top right-hand corner of the compass against the point which represents the landmark and rotate the whole compass until the orienteering lines in the housing are running parallel to the eastings. Draw a line. Repeat the procedure with the second landmark and draw another line. Where the two lines cross is your present position.

GPS (Global Positioning System)

This highly technological and modern method of navigation was first developed by the US Department of Defense. There are 24 military satellites orbiting the Earth, constantly transmitting the time and their location. Anyone with a special receiver can pick up this information, whether they are in the military or not. In fact, since GPS systems entered the civilian market their popularity has grown immensely, especially amongst pilots, sailors and walkers. The GPS receiver unit itself is generally no larger than a mobile phone and is powered by battery. It is able to receive and collate the information from the satellites into useful information, such as grid reference and altitude. In fact, you can find out your location no matter where you are in the world. However, there is generally a built-in fault in the civilian units that makes them a little less accurate than the military ones, which can pinpoint a location within 15 metres or less.

How GPS works

For a GPS unit to work, it needs to be able to locate and receive information from at least four of the orbiting satellites, although the more it can pick up, the better. By a process called satellite ranging, the satellite is able to calculate your position in relation to a number of known objects. The transmitted data is then turned into usable information such as longitude and latitude, 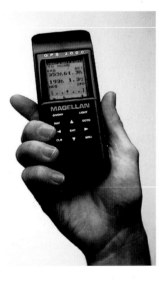 height above sea level and a grid reference. Your position can be updated, as can your speed and track while on the move. To aid with route planning, it can also identify future way-points. Individual needs can be programmed in, making it flexible whether at sea, on land or in the air.

SELECTING A ROUTE

As you are not actually participating in SAS Selection, you have the advantage of choosing your own route. In doing so you can avoid many of the pitfalls which lie in wait for the soldiers, such as bogs, rivers, fences and forests. Additionally, you can make your route circular so that you can arrive back at your transport. The first thing to do is to consult guide books at the local library or talk to a member of a hill walking club such as the Ramblers' Association. Either of these will give you some information on established walks in your area. If you wish, you can purchase an Ordnance Survey map from which you can select your own route. However, there are several factors to bear in mind.

Distance

The distance of your route should not exceed those examples shown in this book, that is, start off by walking a distance of 5 miles (8 kilometres) and extend this to 10 miles (16 kilometres) as you become more proficient.

Terrain

Study the terrain over which you must walk. If you intend leaving a clearly marked footpath and going cross country, make sure you can navigate or read a map and understand the map symbols in the legend. There's nothing wrong with a little hill climbing, but you will find contouring around them much easier. Avoid bogs, crops, thick forests or anything that will bar your way. Do not cross rivers or streams which are more than a foot (30cm) deep.

Way-points

Way-points are used to guide your path from place to place by establishing a recognizable feature. Clearly define the start and finish point of your route. In between make way-points using prominent objects, such as road junctions, bridges and telephone boxes.

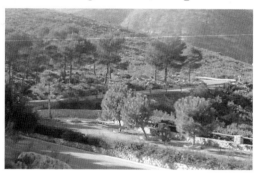

If you are using a pre-published route card, read and understand the details given. Make sure you know your whereabouts at all points along the route.

Make your way-points prominent features of the landscape, such as this sharp bend in the road, which are recognisable on both the map and the ground

Time and Distance

Time and distance are both important individual factors, yet your aim should be to bring the two together at a point where you feel most comfortable while achieving the best results. In the initial stages of your exercise programme the time you spend running is far more important than the distance. Get used to running for a certain time and try to increase the distance by simply running faster.

It is best to start off with a minimum time of 30 minutes. Run at a pace you feel comfortable with, which, ideally, should be between 65 to 75 per cent of your heart rate's maximum capacity. If you need to slow down then do so, or if you feel you could do a little more then that's also fine. The important factor at this level is duration, or put another way, time spent increasing the heart rate.

As you improve your running fitness, measure the distance of your routes and time yourself. At this stage simply time yourself while running normally and do not try to set any records.

THE WEATHER

The weather in the British Isles is unpredictable at best and this is doubly so on hilltops and mountains. Weather can cause many problems and potential dangers for hillwalkers, so you must be aware of sudden changes at all times and be prepared to act accordingly. Although we cannot change the weather, we can to a certain extent predict it.

Before undertaking any hillwalking trip, the weather forecast for the region should be checked. If extreme weather conditions are likely, which are liable to cause exposure and frostbite or heat-stroke, then you should postpone your activity. Always use common sense and try to interpret prevailing weather conditions in the light of the most up-to-date forecast. This becomes even more important in winter. Fatalities which occur as a result of the weather often involve some human carelessness or ignorance; both can be avoided. If the worst happens and you do find yourself and your party trapped on a hill or mountain in bad weather, find shelter, keep together and sit it out. As long as clothing and food are adequate and morale is high, you will stand a good chance of survival. You should be aware that the weather can pose a whole range of problems for the hillwalker.

Heavy rain can cause streams to become fast and swollen. Trying to negotiate a swollen stream is risky to say the least, and potentially life-threatening. Find another route if necessary to detour around it.

Fog can be dangerous as it is disorientating and hides obstacles and hazards, such as cliffs. In such conditions in dangerous terrain you are best advised to stay put until the visibility improves. If you have to keep going, consider roping the members of the party together. In this way you can be assured that no one will get lost and it may also save someone from a nasty fall. Wind gusts, especially in exposed places such as a high ridge-line, can be so powerful as to knock a person off their feet. If there is any danger of this, get all party members to crawl on their hands and knees and keep them close together. Again, it may be necessary to rope everyone together.

Hailstones can be up to 2 cm (1 in) in diameter and rain down with sufficient force to cause serious injury. In the rare event of being caught out in a hailstorm, make sure you find shelter or at least cover your head. It is wise to take precautions against lightning while hillwalking. However, it is very rare for an electrical storm to occur without some advance warning. The appearance of thunderclouds in the distance followed by flashes of lightning and rumbles of thunder are all good indicators. Watch the direction in which the clouds are moving. Note that lightning strikes the easiest point with which to make contact, which is usually the highest point in the area. If you are caught out in a lightning storm, it is much safer to stay out in the open, even if it is in driving rain. Sit down, preferably on your rucksack, and minimize your contact points with the ground by drawing your knees up and placing your hands in your lap.

AUTHOR'S NOTE

➤ I have found a method of anticipating any immediate danger the weather may pose. A clear sky with high cloud will indicate a clear and sunny day. Dark sky with low cloud normally indicates rain. It is simply a matter of gauging the degree between the two. I do this by looking towards my direction of travel and try to estimate the height of cloud, colour of sky and wind direction. With a little practice one is able to anticipate the weather conditions for several hours ahead

Weather Forecasts

In addition to the national television, radio and newspaper weather forecasts, hillwalkers have access to a number of other forecasting services. Weathercall offers forecasts by telephone or by fax. For instance, to get a regional telephone forecast for northwest Scotland, you should ring 0891 500 425, for north Wales 0891 500 415 and for the Lake District 0891 500 419. Similarly, fax forecasts are available for these areas by typing 0897 300 1, plus the appropriate suffix (northwest Scotland is 25), into the fax machine. Weathercall also provides a national seven-day forecast by phone on 0891 500 400. Regional long-range forecasts are also available.

There are also specialized weather forecasts for hillwalkers. BBC Radio Scotland has a daily forecast at 6.55 pm (weekdays) and 6.05 pm (weekends), and in winter this includes an avalanche risk assessment as well. ClimbLine provides regional forecasts for the Western Highlands of Scotland on 0891 333 198 and the Eastern Highlands on 0891 333 197. Most youth hostels in mountainous areas get a faxed daily forecast from the Met Office.

CHECKLIST FOR WINTER WALKING

➤ Check the weather forecast before setting off.

➤ Consult a local guide or expert about the route you intend to follow.

➤ Plan your route with care.

➤　　　Leave a copy of your route with a responsible person.

➤　　　Have a cut-off time for your return.

➤　　　Do not walk alone.

➤　　　Dress using the layer principle (see p.000). Salopettes are warmer than trousers for winter walking. You should protect your hands and head withthermal gloves, a neck-over and a balaclava.

➤　　　Wear comfortable walking boots which are appropriate for winter use.

➤　　　Wear gaiters to protect your boots and lower legs.

➤　　　The amount of calories in the food you carry should be twice that for a summer walk.

➤　　　Remember to carry a flask of hot soup, as portable cookers do not work well in wintry conditions.

➤　　　Watch where you walk.

➤　　　Keep a careful watch on the weather.

➤　　　If you get into trouble, retrace your steps or walk towards the nearest point of known safety.

SAMPLE ROUTES

The following sample routes are designed to help you come to terms with the concept of SAS Selection. You do not have to travel to the Brecon Beacons to walk these routes, moreover you should endeavour to find somewhere near to home and select similar routes of your own. Don't forget you are only training and putting into practice all the points mentioned above.

Carry a light load (22 lbs –10 kg – max.) and include in this protective clothing, an emergency kit and a light snack. Pace yourself going up hill and jog carefully going downhill to avoid injury. Before you set off leave details of your intended route with someone. The timings shown are based on averaging roughly 16 minutes per kilometre over terrain similar to the Brecon Beacons.

The purpose of the following is to help you select and set your own routes, improve your map reading and so prepare you for the extreme fitness programme. While you are encouraged to time your route, finishing is the main goal. I would recommend that you complete no more than two routes per week.

You should obtain a copy of Ordnance Survey map 1:50,000 Landranger Series Sheet 160 to study the sample routes detailed.

Route 1

This is designed to be a simple map-reading route, starting at one place and finishing at another, and along the way passing through a number of easily recognizable way-points. When selecting a similar route yourself I would advise that you try to avoid difficult or dangerous terrain, and make sure you have a lift waiting for you at the finish.

ROUTE 1

Walking distance: approx. 9 miles (15 km)

Time: 4–5 hours

Dress: equipped for the outdoors;
rucksack weight 10 lbs (4.5 kg): warm-up

1 Start at GR896222 where the small track runs
   southeast from the B-class road. Follow the track
   as it turns south following it until you are halfway
   around the forest at Bwleh-y-Duwynt. At this
   point take a compass bearing on the dam end of
   Yetradfelle Reservoir, GR945174, and make your
   own way across country.
2 Upon arrival at Yetradfelle Reservoir take a new
   bearing heading for the road junction at the
   southern end of Beacons Reservoir, GR989182.

Route 2

The idea behind Route 2 is to draw a sketch map,
which will force you to use your compass, walking
from point to point by dead reckoning. This is
simply achieved by blotting out the bulk of the map
detail leaving just a small patch surrounding each

way-point. My advice is to make your own sketch map using short distances to start with, and then build up to a 5 or 6 kilometres separation. Time and distance are really important, as is recognizing the main feature you are heading for. Sketch maps are designed to aid navigation during poor visibility.

ROUTE 2

Walking distance: approx. 11 miles (18 km)

Time: 5–6 hours

Dress: equipped for the outdoors;

rucksack weight 10 lbs (4.5 kg); warm-up

1 Start at any of the five points and make your way around them. Each of the areas is in its precise position, making bearings and distance accurate.

2 A: a small road junction at the edge of the forest.

3 B: where a gate leads to a forest track (the stream is not there, but the ground is boggy).

4 C: a river bridge – make sure you get the correct one as there are several near by.

5 D: a river junction in the forest, very easy to find.

6 E: a pool on the edge of a golf course.

AUTHOR'S NOTE

➤ The easiest way to make a sketch map is
to place an A4 sheet of paper over the
map. Next, using a ten-pence piece, or
similar, draw five circles at equal
distances apart and cut them out. Lay the
paper on top of a map and photocopy
and you have one sketch map. Always
take a proper map of the area with you,
but only use it if you get completely lost.

Route 3

This is the longest route and is designed to test not
just your map-reading ability but also your stamina. It
uses a main hill feature as the centre point around
which the route climbs and descends several times.
This helps you concentrate your efforts on improving
your overall time.

You should continue practising route planning and
map reading until you feel confident enough to
participate in the final programme. You will need to
have completed at least 10 to 15 such routes before
embarking on such a rigorous course.

ROUTE 3

Walking distance: approx. 16 miles (26 km)

Time: 5–8 hours

Dress: equipped for the outdoors;
rucksack weight 20 lbs (9 kg); warm-up

1 Start at the car park just south of Cwmgwdi,
   GR024249, which is situated by the old army
   camp. Make your way uphill, heading south-
   southwest, to Twyn Cil-rhew, staying with the
   main track and continuing along the ridge up to
   Pen-y-Fan, GR012215. You cannot miss it, it's the
   highest feature in the Beacons range and very
   prominent on a clear day. Be very careful as you
   get close to the top, the northern edge turns into
   a sheer escarpment.

2 From Pen-y-Fan continue walking southwest
   around Corn Du, dropping down the very prominent track to the car park, GR987198 – 1000 m
   south of the Story Arms.

3 Retrace your footsteps back up to Pen-y-Fan turn-

ing east at the trig-point 886 dropping down the steep slope onto the track that contours south of the Graig Cwm Cynwyn ridgeline to point 599, GR032205. From here walk directly south along Tor Glas until you reach the road/track junction at GR035174.

4 Retrace your footsteps back up to Pen-y-Fan, turning north-northeast back down to the car park at Cwmgwdi.

You can do this route from any of the other points, but the Story Arms offers a good starting point as there are toilets and refreshments available – the other locations are accessible but isolated.

SAFETY

If you are new to hillwalking and have no practical knowledge of map reading, I suggest you start by following the more scenic routes, which are clearly marked and frequently used by other walkers. Almost all the good walks in Great Britain, Europe and America have been well documented in a wide variety of books that are readily available. These will provide a map showing details of the route and will also indicate distance.

As with all forms of activity, basic safety rules must be observed. If you intend to walk in an isolated area then any injury or illness that incapacitates you becomes a very serious problem. Therefore you must be prepared.

SAFETY PRECAUTIONS

➤ Whenever possible walk or run your routes in the company of others.

➤ If alone stick to those routes frequented by others and leave full details of your route and timings with someone trustworthy.

➤ Carry a mobile phone and have the emergency numbers for the police, rescue services, etc. stuck on the back.

➤ Always carry a map and compass or route card so that you can indicate your location.

➤ Dress and carry equipment to suit the prevailing weather conditions.

➤ Check the weather conditions before you start off.

FINISHING

The aim of these routes is to get fit enough to try out for the SAS Selection. Unlike the SAS soldiers who must complete a given distance in a given time, however, you have no need to rush. Start off by warming up properly and try to avoid routes which go directly into a hill climb. If this is the case, tackle them at a slow pace, keeping your breathing under control. If you start to feel tired, slow down but avoid stopping. If, on the other hand, you feel the need for a little jog along a flat or slight decline then do so. The idea is to reach a point whereby you enjoy walking along, feeling the freedom of the hills and the beauty of nature. When you have completed your route give yourself a little treat: go to the pub with your companions and talk over your accomplishment. Check and note your timings, be critical of any mistakes and praise your efforts. Most of all, relax and soak in the feeling of euphoric fitness.

WARNING

➤ The longest hillwalking exercise described here is six hours, so there is no need to sleep out overnight. However, weather conditions can change quickly and it is wise to take precautions.

SAS Selection Techniques

This chapter deals with a series of routes taken while on SAS Selection. If you decide to become super-fit and have prepared yourself properly, you can match your endurance in a similar way to the soldier on SAS Selection. The full programme runs for 17 days, and although soldiers are required to perform non-stop, you have the option of breaking the routes down into a series of weekend activities.

SAS Selection takes place in the Brecon Beacons, South Wales, but as most people will not have access to them they should be used as a guide to make up your own routes. To do this with reasonable accuracy,

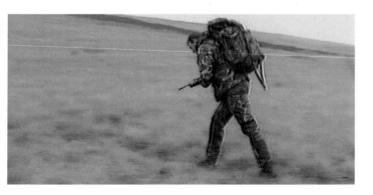

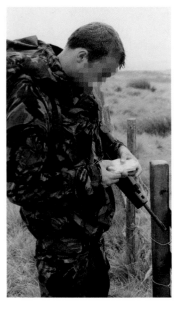

the area over which you select your routes should be similar in terrain. The Brecon Beacons are not a high range of mountains, but they are treacherous. Exposed and battered by constant weather changes, death by hypothermia is seldom far away for the potential SAS soldiers, and over the years many have suffered this slow death. For the purpose of route selection the British Isles provides many such similar areas to the Brecon Beacons, such as Dartmoor, Snowdonia, the Peak District, Yorkshire Dales and the Lake District. Mid- and North Scotland also provide a whole host of mountainous areas, and all with the added benefit of outstanding scenery.

However, these areas can be equally as dangerous as the Brecon Beacons during bad weather. The build-up training dealt with the basics of good navigation, now we need to know how to equip ourselves properly for walking outdoors.

HILLWALKING EQUIPMENT

Before beginning the next stage of the fitness programme you must make certain preparations. The outdoors can be unpredictable and even dangerous in certain conditions and you will need to ensure that you are properly dressed and equipped. Having the right kind of clothes is especially important to protect the body from the effects of weather. A person's functioning body temperature is usually between 96°F and 102°F. If the body temperature falls outside either of these then vital functions will begin to come under strain and will eventually fail, often leading to death. It is vital that the correct body temperature is maintained, no matter what the weather conditions, otherwise serious complications could occur.

There are many external factors which play a part in affecting the temperature of the body: air temperature; wet; loss of moisture; wind; illness; injury and shock. Body heat can either be leached or added to by the processes of convection, conduction and radiation. However, one of the biggest problems in any outdoor situation is the wind, because it can worsen any situation. If the air temperature is cold and the body wet, the addition of a wind causes an extra chilling factor, taking away vital reserves of body heat and cooling the core temperature of the body too quickly. This will soon cause death. Just as deadly, a wind operating in hot, dry conditions will deplete the body of essential moisture.

Weather can be unpredictable, changing from a hot day to a gale or even a snowstorm within hours. This is especially true in certain climates and also at altitude. Emergencies may occur at any time, so it is always best to be prepared for the worst, so that there is a greater chance that you will survive. In order to protect our body's core temperature you must make sure that you wear the correct protective clothing at all times.

OVERHEATING AND SWEATING

You may be surprised to know that it is possible to get heat exhaustion even when the weather is freezing. This can be caused by exertion while wearing too many layers of clothing. Heat is evenly distributed around the body by the blood, therefore any area in which the bloodflow becomes restricted will soon suffer either from too much heat or not enough. The biggest culprit in restricting bloodflow is tight clothing, especially cuffs around the wrists, ankles, waist and neck. Gloves and socks, too, may cause discomfort and overheating. Always make sure if you're wearing two layers that the outer one is large enough to fit comfortably over the inner one.

At the first sign of overheating act accordingly. Loosen clothing at the neck, wrists and waist to allow a little more air and blood to circulate. If you still find that you're not cooling down enough, start to remove your outer layers of clothing, but do it one layer at a time. Of course, as soon as you stop overheating replace the layers again so that your body does not get chilled. If you need to remove layers when the weather is wet, do not remove any waterproof outer layer, but instead take off one of the inner layers.

How the Layer System Works

One way of controlling body temperature is by using a layer system of clothing. This method depends on lots of thin layers rather than just one or two thick garments. Air gets trapped between the layers and warmed, providing insulation and protection from loss of body heat. The temperature can also be easily controlled by either adding or removing layers.

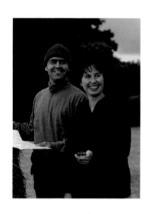

The clothes that you wear next to your skin should be comfortable, loose-fitting, light and preferably made of cotton; for example, a thermal cotton vest would be ideal. As this layer lies closest to the skin it is also the layer which will have to absorb perspiration. It is important, therefore, that underclothes are changed daily and washed.

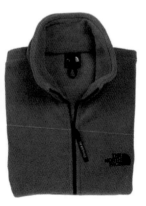

Over the top of the underwear you should wear something that, preferably, can be fastened at the neck and wrists. This will further trap any warm air produced by the body. However, the fastenings should not be so tight as to restrict bloodflow. An ideal sort of garment for this would be a sweater with a zip up collar.

The third layer needs to be a warm, easily removable jacket or over-top. Those made from a fleece-type material would be a good choice.

The last layer should always be one that is windproof and waterproof. There are many coats and jackets on the market which are ideal for this purpose. They tend to be made from nylon, fibre-pile material, tightly woven cotton or polycotton. The best outer garments, however, are those made from Gore-Tex as these also allow any trapped condensation to permeate through the material, thus lessening the chances of both chilling and over-heating. If possible, always choose a coat with a well-fitting hood so that as much of the face and head can be protected as well.

Remember that any exertion, even fast walking, will cause the body to sweat. This sweat will make your clothing wet and will help leach away body warmth. Sweat, also, over time will cause the fibres of the fabric to deteriorate, thus ruining the clothing.

AUTHOR'S NOTE

➤ If you find yourself getting hot while doing anything strenuous, make sure you remove some of your underlayers. Once you stop your activity, replace them again. By getting into this habit you will ensure that you always have a dry layer next to your skin.

HEAD, HANDS AND FEET

The body loses up to a third of
its heat through the head, so
this area is of particular
importance in both hot and
cold climates. Where the
weather is cold, it is important
to protect this area from heat loss by
wearing a scarf or a head-over (a knitted
woollen tube worn around the neck and pulled up
over the head as required). These items are easy to
remove to avoid overheating during strenuous activity.
This head protection should still be worn even if your
outer garment has a waterproof hood attached.

During hot weather, the body can easily overheat if
the head is not covered. Such overheating will lead to
sunstroke, which is a potentially fatal condition. An
unprotected head also risks serious sunburn. To
protect against these possibilities, wear a soft, wide-
brimmed hat.

Apart from the head, the other parts of the body to
suffer most from the cold and wet are the hands and
feet. Both of these are at the extremities of the
circulation and therefore liable to suffer a dangerous
loss of temperature causing unpleasant and life-
threatening conditions, such as frostbite. The best way
to prevent this happening is to avoid getting these
areas wet and cold in the first place. Feet can be
protected by wearing watertight boots and a couple of
layers of socks, although it is important that these

layers do not impede the circulation at all or else the problem will be made worse. In the same way, ensure that the boots are not too tightly laced. The first sign of the bloodflow being hindered is a feeling of numbness, especially in the toes. Check that this is not happening by stopping every now and again and wriggling your toes. If your feet do happen to get wet, make sure that you change your wet socks for some dry ones at the first opportunity you get.

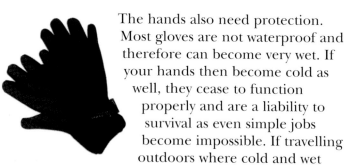

The hands also need protection. Most gloves are not waterproof and therefore can become very wet. If your hands then become cold as well, they cease to function properly and are a liability to survival as even simple jobs become impossible. If travelling outdoors where cold and wet conditions are a possibility, then you should always carry at least one good pair of loose-fitting gloves with you. The warmest types are mittens as these have a greater amount of air circulating around the fingers, however these are not the most practical if you have to use your fingers a lot to carry out tasks. As well as gloves, it is also a good idea to carry a spare pair of socks as these can also be used instead of gloves if the original pair become too wet to be worn.

BOOTS AND FOOTWEAR

Feet work hard, covering long distances and supporting your weight, but it is very easy to ignore them – until they start to hurt or get blisters. The way you look after your feet and the type of footwear you choose is more important than you might think if you are contemplating participating in any kind of outdoor activity. Walking, especially if you are carrying a heavy rucksack, puts a great deal of pressure on the feet. In addition you may also be travelling over rough terrain which will subject them to even more stresses. It is common sense that feet and footwear need to be cared for properly.

Selecting Footwear

Footwear should always be chosen for the purpose in mind. For the sort of training described in this book a pair of walking boots which combine lightness with adequate ankle support and water protection should be sufficient. There are many boots on the market and the number of styles can be very confusing. To add to the complications, a good pair of boots is usually quite expensive and so most people can only afford one pair at a time. It can often be quite daunting when it comes to choosing the right kind of boot.

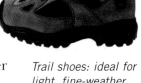

Trail shoes: ideal for light, fine-weather walking

3-season boots: light and stiff-soled for increased protection and support

Some boots are advertised as being designed for climbing over rugged terrain, while others are

4-season boots: warm and rigid, with special lugs on the sole to allow crampons to be fitted

better suited to less arduous walks. There are heavy, waterproofed boots for winter conditions, and lighter, cooler ones for the summer. In the end try to find one that provides the best compromise for all of your needs.

Apart from boots, the choice of socks is also important. Heavier boots will need two pairs of socks: a lightweight inner sock made of wool or silk for warmth, and a thicker outer sock which will act as a cushion for the foot. Lighter boots, made of fabric will need only one pair of socks. There are certain things to consider when buying a new pair of walking boots:

➤   Take and wear the same kind of socks in which you would normally go walking.

➤   When your feet are in the boots, your toes should not touch the ends.

➤   The boot should not feel tight in any area, just comfortable.

➤   Consider the weight and make sure that it is correct for your needs.

➤   Choose a boot that is waterproof.

➤ Make sure that the boot has a well cushioned insole and upper lining, giving firm yet comfortable support to the whole foot.

➤ The backstay, heel corner and toecap should all be strong enough to protect and support the boot.

➤ The boot should come up high enough around the ankle to give it both support and protection. A padded scree collar and a bellows tongue are also a good idea so that the foot is protected against both water and stones.

➤ When trying on the boot, stand on an incline; if you feel that your toes are trapped in the end of the boot, try the next size up.

AUTHOR'S NOTE

➤ Any foot problems such as corns, bunions or ingrown toenails should be treated before you buy any new footwear.

Look at the way the boot was made and consider the maintenance it will need. Fabric boots will not require much more than being kept clean, but leather boots will also need constant applications of wax to keep them supple and watertight. Get a boot with a good grip because this could avoid serious injury, especially if you find yourself on wet and slippery terrain. A rubber star-patterned sole will give you the best grip. PVC will not give much traction at all and is best avoided. Choose a sole thickness in accordance with the sort of terrain you are expecting to walk over. Mountaineering will require a much thicker and stiffer sole than hillwalking. Give the sole a twist to test its flexibility – it should still be solid enough to give good support if you fall.

Footwear Maintenance

New boots should be worn in before going out on any long walks and this may take some time. It is a small price to pay for comfort, however. Begin by wearing them with the laces a little loose and always check that the tongue is flat against the insole of your foot. Start by going on short walks, or even by wearing them around the house. This will enable you to identify any problems before embarking on a long walk.

The boots will need to be looked after carefully if you want them to last. Clean any mud off as soon as you can before washing them. Once clean, they should be polished or sprayed. Wet leather boots will need to be

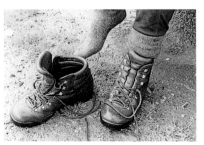

dried carefully as too much direct heat will cause them to crack. First, take out any detachable insoles and wet laces and dry them separately. Second, stuff your boots with something absorbent, such as newspaper or tissues and leave them in a warm place. Once the boots have dried they will need to be treated with several applications of wax or some other water-proofing compound.

RUCKSACKS

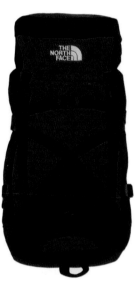

The exercises in this book require that you have a bergen or rucksack large enough to carry all that you need for your walks, as well as items you might need in an emergency situation. These items should include food, water, some kind of shelter, sleeping bag and clothes. Regard your rucksack as a snail would regard its shell: it is your outdoor home, and as such should carry all that you need.

The design of rucksacks has improved remarkably over the years, combining the best of modern technical design and new materials such as two-ply polycotton and Cordura. The rucksacks of today have a high degree of comfort and stability, and come in all shapes and sizes for every kind of outdoor activity. You will need a bergen with a capacity of about 35 litres.

Rucksacks and Weight

Many people who choose their rucksacks wrongly or

go for the cheapest options end up with backache, or, even worse, a badly strained back. The spinal column acts as a support for the whole of the upper body, transferring weight down onto the pelvic bones. It is a triumph of engineering in its own right and is constructed as a series of curves which allow for the absorbence of shocks as well as giving the body a good degree of flexibility. The largest of these curves is found in the lower back and is known as the lordosis. This is the part of the spine most designed to take any strain, due to its spring-like construction. Accordingly, this is also the area that is most vulnerable to backache.

When choosing a rucksack bear the above in mind and make sure that it fits in with your body shape, preferably with a wide, padded waistbelt as this will take some of the weight off the spine and transfer it straight to the hips. The centre of gravity of the pack should be high on your back, with the rest of the weight evenly distributed between your shoulders and your hips. This will ensure that instead of the back doing all the work, your legs will also help to bear the weight. When the rucksack is full, make sure that it is able to support the weight in a stable manner.

Fitting your Pack

Packing a rucksack correctly is an art and one that should

be learned before you go out into the field. First, you need to know what to pack so that unnecessary items are left at home, not adding to the weight on your back. Second, you should be sure that once everything is packed you can still get at anything you want with a minimum of effort.

Side pockets are the easiest to get to and therefore should hold things you will need while you are walking, such as water, flasks and snacks. These pockets are also useful for carrying Camel hydration systems (a tube and water container set-up that allows the walker to drink without having to stop). Coats and items of clothing needed if the weather turns nasty should be neatly folded beneath the top flap of your rucksack. The bergen itself should be packed with items used less frequently, such as a sleeping bag, at the bottom, and those you are likely to use more often at the top.

SAS SELECTION ROUTES

The following 18-day fitness course is designed around the early exercise tests encountered while doing SAS Selection. However, in addition to their rucksacks the participating soldiers will be expected to carry a rifle and a 15-lb (7-kg) belt kit. The sample routes are based on those covered by the SAS and should be used as a guide to plan similar routes in your chosen area.

Food consumption during this 18-day course is unlimited with the suggestion that you plan a high protein and carbohydrate diet. Not that you will feel like drinking alcohol but you should abstain altogether during the course.

SAS ACTION

➤ Sometimes in the SAS it seems that you are forever walking attached to your bergen. This seems to start with Selection and then continues throughout your service. Therefore if anyone knows how to pack a bergen, an SAS soldier does. Before every operation he will scrutinize the contents of his pack, taking out anything that will be unnecessary and therefore add to the weight. This also sometimes means a bit of improvisation: throwing away any excess food wrappings and even taking food out of tins and repackaging it in plastic bags. Luxuries are a complete non-starter. When it comes down to it, you should be able to put your rucksack on your back and then forget about it as you walk. If it is too heavy or unbalanced, this will not be possible and you will find the walk an awful experience.

The course has two sets of rest days spaced at five-day intervals. You should use the rest days to relax, treat any medical problems, eat and sleep.

DAY ONE

Dress: equipped for outdoors
Rucksack weight: 30 lbs (14 kg)

Morning:

Warm-up. Find a suitable road and complete the following fitness test. You will need a friend to assist you in some of the exercises.

5-km run; fireman's lift 100 m; 20 push-ups;
baby carry 200 m; 2-mile walk

Afternoon:

Find a steep hill of at 100 m.
Warm-up, then complete 20 x 100 m up the hill.

No time limit.

DAY TWO

Dress: equipped for outdoors
Rucksack weight: 40 lbs (18 kg)

Fan Dance
Warm-up. Find a mountainous peak of around 1000 m above sea level and choose three points around the peak at a distance of around 3 miles

(5 km). Total distance 15 miles (24 km).

Sample route:
Start-point lay-by grid 987198 ➤ RV1 Pen-y-Fan grid 012 216 ➤ RV2 Track junction 033 182 ➤ RV3 Pen-y-Fan grid 012 216 ➤ RV4 Road / bridge junction grid 985241 ➤ RV5 Pen-y-Fan grid 012 216 ➤ finish-/start-point grid 987198

Complete the distance inside 6 hours.

DAY THREE

Dress: equipped for outdoors
Rucksack weight: no rucksack required

Beasting
Warm-up. Find a short flat deserted road or track. You will require the services of a friend about your own weight. Complete the following in under 1 hour:

Firemans-lift 200m; 20 push-ups; baby carry 200m; 20 push-ups; piggy-back ride 200m; 20 push-ups; fireman's lift 200m;

20 push-ups; baby carry 200m; 20 push-ups; piggy-back 200m; 20 push-ups.

Afternoon:
Locate a steep hill of at least 200 metres. Warm-up. Complete 20 x 200 m up the hill.

DAY FOUR

Dress: equipped for outdoors
Rucksack weight: 40 lbs (18 kg)

Warm-up. Swimming test: 20 circuits of the local swimming pool. Tread water for 10 minutes.

Afternoon:

Map-reading exercise: sample route – start-point road/lay-by grid 0175 1060 ➤ RV1 bridge grid 9450 1120 ➤ RV2 pot-hole grid 8910 1615 ➤ finish-point road junction grid 844 164.

No time limit.

DAYS FIVE AND SIX

Rest days.

DAY SEVEN

Dress: equipped for outdoors
Rucksack weight: 30 lbs (14 kg)

Warm-up. Map-reading exercise number 2: choose a hilly area some 11 miles (18 km) in distance.

Sample route – start-point road/stream junction grid 967126 ➤ RV1 Yetradfelle reservoir grid 944 073 ➤ RV2 road/stream junction grid 926208 ➤ finish-point lay-by grid 855179.

Time taken 5 hours.

DAY EIGHT

Dress: equipped for outdoors
Rucksack weight: 40 lbs (18 kg)

Warm-up. Map-reading exercise number 3: choose a route about 9 miles (15 km) in distance over lowland forested terrain. Sample route: start-point road junction grid 1080 6465 ➤ RV1 trig-point 538 grid 1705 6065 ➤ RV2 east end of pool grid 1400 5940 ➤ RV3 telephone box grid 1255 5820 ➤ finish-point road/ river bridge grid 1140 5445

Time taken 4 hours 30 minutes.

DAY NINE

Dress: equipped for outdoors
Rucksack weight: 40 lbs (18 kg)

Warm-up. Map-reading exercise number 4: choose a route about 12 miles (20 km) in distance over lowland forested terrain. Sample route: start-point pub car park grid 8810 2915 ➤ RV1 standing stones grid 8335 2835 ➤ RV2 standing stones grid 8360 2570 ➤ RV3 spot-height 591 grid 8475 2315 ➤ RV4 spot-height 562 grid 8620 2065 ➤ RV5 spot-height 582 grid 9080 2640 ➤ finish-/start-point grid 8810 2915

Time taken 4 hours 30 minutes.

DAY TEN

Dress: equipped for outdoors
Rucksack weight: 40 lbs (18 kg)

Warm-up. Map-reading exercise number 5: choose a route about 81/2 miles (14 km) in distance over hill and forested terrain. Sample route: start-point telephone box grid 172 585 ➤ RV1 spot-height 523 grid 193 609 ➤ RV2 trig-point 660 grid 182 639 ➤ RV3 spot-height 491 grid 159 635 ➤ RV4 trig-point 538 grid 171 606 ➤ finish-/start-point grid 172 585

Time taken 4 hours.

DAY ELEVEN

Dress: equipped for outdoors
Rucksack : 45 lbs (20 kg)

Warm-up. Map reading exercise number 6: choose a route about 18 miles (29 km) in distance over mixed hill and forested terrain. Sample route: start-point road junction grid 160 647 ➤ RV1 spot-height 491 grid 159 635 ➤ RV2 AA box grid 198 598 ➤ RV3 trig-point 610 grid 214 636 ➤ RV4 stream junction grid 202 671 ➤ Finish-/start-point grid 160 647

Time taken 6 hours.

DAYS TWELVE AND THIRTEEN

Rest days.

DAY FOURTEEN

Dress: equipped for outdoors
Rucksack weight: 50 lbs (23 kg)

Pipeline

Warm-up. Choose a route about 14 miles (23 km) in distance over steep hills. Sample route: start-point lay-by near dam grid 987 198 ‰ RV1 spot-height 632 grid 938 186 ‰ RV2 pot-hole grid 891 161 ‰ RV3 trig-point 725 grid 881 191 ‰ RV4 trig-point 603 grid 912 216 ä RV5 spot-height 632 grid 938 186 ‰ finish-/startpoint grid 987 198.

Time taken 5 hours 30 minutes

DAY FIFTEEN

Dress: equipped for outdoors
Rucksack weight: 50 lbs (23 kg)

Point to Point

Choose a route about 25 km in distance over steep hills. Sample route: start-point lay-by grid 972 222 ➤ RV1 Pen-y-Fan grid 012 216 ➤ RV2 car park grid 024 249 ➤ RV3 Pen-y-Fan grid 012 216 ➤ RV4 track junction grid 034 182 ➤ RV5 Pen-y-Fan grid 012 216 ➤ finish-/start-point grid 972 222

Time taken 6 hours.

DAY SIXTEEN

Dress: equipped for outdoors
Rucksack weight: 70 lbs (32 kg)

Heavy Carry

Choose a route about 9 miles (15 km) in distance over steep hills. Sample route: start-point road junction grid 773 259 ➤ RV1 stone circle grid 808 244 ➤ RV2 trig-point 802 grid 826 218 ➤ finish-point road junction grid 861 246

Time 4 hours 30 minutes.

DAY SEVENTEEN

Dress: equipped for outdoors
Rucksack weight: 55 lbs (25 kg)

Endurance

Choose a route about 40 miles (65 km) in distance over steep hills. Sample route: start-point road junction grid 080 260 ➤ RV1 track junction grid 034 182 ➤ RV2 Fan Fawr grod 964 189 ➤ RV3 trig-point 603 grid 912 216 ➤ RV4 road / track junction grid 868 193 ➤ RV5 Yetradfelle reservoir grid 944 073 ➤ RV6 road bridge grid 995 164 ➤ RV7 track junction grid 034 183 ➤ finish-point grid 080 260

Time taken 20 hours.

Complete the course within the times and you should be proud of yourself. Completion within an hour of the times is also good and still gives you something to aim for.

Fitness Health and Injuries

AVOIDING INJURY

A medical chapter in a fitness book may at first seem strange, but the reasons for its inclusion will soon become apparent. For a start it serves as a warning not to exercise while overweight or seriously unfit. This can damage a body that is unused to exertion. In the worst case it could lead to a heart attack. Even in a fit person, exercise can still cause injury if that person is not careful about the way he uses his body.

This chapter aims to focus on the risks and medical problems associated with getting fit and exploring the great outdoors. It is one thing getting a sprain or blisters either at home or in the gym, but if you sustain the same injury while walking out alone in remote areas with the weather closing in, it could be a matter of life and death. This is not to say that the potential dangers should put you off: the advantages of exercising still far outweigh any risks. However, there is nothing wrong with being aware that something might just go awry, and knowing what you can do about it. It is wise to be prepared.

Intense exercising will often cause injuries as the body is pushed beyond its normal limits. However, with a sensible training regime it should be possible to minimize any risk and stay safe. A well-balanced exercise programme will always include a warm-up and cool down, will never place too much stress on any one part of the body, and will allow time for recovery. If any part of your body has a weakness, start off by strengthening it with gentle exercises; stretching will limit the possibility of damage. Run or jog on a smooth, level surface to avoid sprains and strains. Bear in mind that most problems are caused by overusing a muscle or a joint, exercising too much or too intensely without time for the body to recover.

If, despite taking every precaution, you find that you have injured yourself, stop what you are doing immediately and seek medical help. Carrying on will only make it worse, whereas an injury that is treated straight away will stand a better chance of healing quickly. Most injuries caused by overuse can be treated with RICE – rest, ice, compression and elevation. Injuries are generally caused by:

➤ Being overweight or too unfit while exercising.
➤ Training too hard and too quickly.
➤ Playing in a high-contact sport such as rugby.
➤ Hard surfaces.
➤ Addiction to exercise (where it becomes the be-all and end-all of your life).
➤ Traffic accidents (this applies mainly to roadrunners and cyclists).

Training while Unfit or Overweight

This subject has been well covered, however, it is wise to remember the repercussions. Pushing your body into a series of strenuous exercises while grossly overweight or unfit can produce a heart attack. The only way to approach fitness safely is to lose weight and exercise slowly. Apart from physical injury, such as a strain or broken bone, you should also be aware of other symptoms during exercise, such as :

➤ Severe chest pain
➤ Sudden headache
➤ Abdominal pain
➤ Dizziness
➤ Nausea and vomiting
➤ Severe pain to the body without obvious physical reason

Always take prompt action. Stop exercising and rest. If the symptoms continue or reoccur after exercise is resumed then seek immediate medical assistance.

Training too hard

While enthusiasm is a great motivator, exercising beyond your current physical condition will only produce a negative affect. As any marathon runner will tell you, there is a point at which the body is totally drained of energy; to exercise beyond this point will cause muscle fatigue. Always exercise so that the body's aerobic system is functioning at around 75–80 per cent of capacity.

Contact Injuries

We are not all inclined to take
up walking as a form of fitness.
Some people prefer more social
sports such as football, martial
arts or bike riding. The
problem here is contact.
Contact when tackled by
another player, contact when

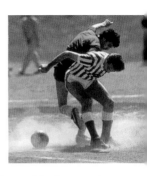

your opponent hits you with a miss-guided punch, or
when a dog runs in front of you and you fall off your
bike, making contact with the road.

Traffic Accidents

Accidents on the road involving joggers and cyclists
are not that frequent but can be very serious.
Avoidance is the best defence against a road traffic
accident. Jog or walk on tracks not used by vehicles.
Don't wear headphones while running on the road.
Wear light or reflective clothing during the hours of
dusk and darkness.

Training on a Hard Surface

Running on hard surfaces causes
many leg injuries, especially in the
knee. Avoid running on hard road
surfaces or concrete. Soft, even
surfaces are best for injury
prevention. Whenever possible,
run on grass or dirt paths, or in
parks. However, if hard surface
running is all that is available to

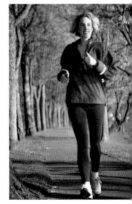

you, make sure you exercise with appropriate footwear for the conditions, and allow extra recovery periods.

FITNESS OBSESSION AND OVER-TRAINING

For those that start a fitness programme it seems silly to think that they may reach the point at which they are over-training. That first walk or jog you take burns your chest, forces you to breathe at an accelerated rate while muscles refuse to function – at this stage it seems unlikely that over-training will ever be a problem. However, some people as they get fitter will come to relish their newfound ability and concentrate on their fitness to the point where it becomes an obsession. It must be stressed that all forms of training and exercising must be done at a set pace and in balance with the body's resources. If you push yourself too hard for too long, you will begin to feel fatigued. Over-training will do very little to improve your fitness. We all have good days where we want to continue training well past our allocated period, likewise we all has bad days when we don't want to leave the house, never mind go to the gym.

Not surprisingly the signs of over-training are very similar to those of stress. There is a loss of appetite, insomnia, lack of concentration, irritability and frequent injury. The mental ability to recognize these signs is vital and they are easy to detect, as your body screams at you for a break or to find some alternative. You know if you are training too hard, because instead of improvement and a general feeling of well-

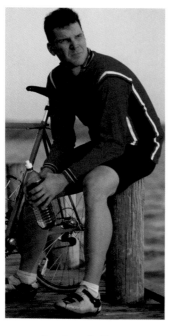

being, you feel like you did before you started your fitness programme. Likewise, if your training partner, if you have one, says that you are overdoing it, you must listen to them.

The best cure for over-training is to take a break, relax and do nothing for at least two weeks. This will give both your body and mind time to readjust. Recovery from exercise fatigue requires total rest and an increased diet. All forms of fitness should be suspended until your appetite has fully returned and the body has reverted to its normal balance. Stress and poor diet will only prolong the fatigue.

After two weeks your should find both your body and mind more relaxed, to the point where you are feeling, eating and sleeping better. If you can not force yourself into a period of inactivity, and many find it difficult, then choose a totally different form of exercise, e.g, if you where on an aerobic routine, change to a muscle programme and vice versa. This will slow down your body for a short while but will still prove beneficial. If you take this later course, you must improve your calorie intake to help compensate

AUTHOR'S NOTE

➤ An ex-military friend of mine who is now employed as a gym teacher set himself the goal of running a 5-day marathon across the Saudi Arabian desert. At the age of 59 this would have been a major achievement. He trained exceptionally hard – too hard. On the fourth day of the race he became sluggish and floundered, unable to carry on. He had pushed himself too hard during training. Upon his return to England he was a different man, fatigue had set in which had totally demoralized him.

TYPICAL INJURIES

Certain injuries are more commonly associated with exercise than others. These are:

➤ Chafing (abrasions caused either by skin rubbing against skin or material rubbing against skin)

➤ Broken bones, dislocations or displacement of one or more bones in a joint

➤ Blisters

➤ Sprains and muscle strains

➤ Back injuries

➤ Shinsplints

Shinsplints

These are injuries caused to the shinbones and the soft tissues in that area. They are generally caused by running on hard surfaces without good shock protection or wearing shoes with rigid soles. Running or walking on the balls of the feet will also cause this painful injury.

Your Feet

Without feet many of the exercises in this book, such as the hillwalking, jogging and running, could not be done. That is why it is so important that the feet are cared for. For instance, ingrown toenails and blisters should be treated as soon as they occur, otherwise they will only get more painful and end up delaying or even preventing you continuing with the exercise programme.

Blisters

Blisters on a foot are something that most people have experienced at some time in their life. They are usually caused by footwear that doesn't fit properly, socks of poor quality or loose laces. In addition to these, having to walk long distances over rough terrain, especially

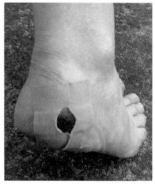

if the foot becomes wet, will cause blisters to develop.

In general, blisters are not serious and can be treated

as a minor injury. However, the pain they cause can often be so bad as to be disabling and this will be disastrous if out on a long walk and a good way from home. To avoid getting blisters, make sure that your footwear fits well and is well worn in before attempting any long excursions. Also, make sure that your feet are kept clean and dry.

Blisters should be treated the moment they appear; to leave them longer will create a sore that may become infected and slow to heal. As soon as you feel a sore spot, stop, put some antiseptic cream on it and cover it with a plaster or a surgical dressing, making sure there are no creases in the tape. Micropore tape can be used on the toes. If a fluid-filled blister is already present, use a blister ring instead. This will protect the area against any further pressure.

A large fluid-filled blister will often be extremely uncomfortable. The pressure can be relieved by draining the fluid. Do not do this by bursting it, as this will only expose an area of raw skin underneath and leave it open to infection. Wash the foot thoroughly first and then sterilize a needle. Prick the blister at the bottom edge and then gently press out the fluid, taking as much time as it needs. Once this has been done, cover the area with a blister ring. This should be changed every day and the area cleansed each time. Blisters can be helped to heal by immersing the foot in a hot, salty footbath.

However, make sure that you dry off the area around the blister thoroughly – blisters need to be clean and dry to heal.

SAS ACTION

➤ One survival method of relieving the pressure from an ingrown toenail is to shave the top centre of the nail with a safety razor blade. Skim the middle third of the nail, shaving from the bed towards the nail-tip. Place a thin piece of plastic under the nail to prevent any accidental cutting of the toe front. When the nail is thin enough it will buckle into a ridge and relieve the outer pressure. Removing the nail altogether should be avoided, as this will require a dressing and may prevent exercise for several weeks.

Ingrown Toenails

Ingrown toenails are caused when the nail grows into the flesh at the sides of the toe, leading to severe pain and infection. They are painful enough to prevent exercise, and should be treated as

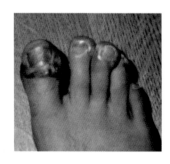

soon as they are detected. Initially, by cutting a 'V' down the centre of the nail this will help relieve the pain and may cure the problem. However, if the toe has become infected you are advised to see a chiropodist or your doctor for treatment at once, because the nail will most probably need removing.

Corns

These are painful pads of thick hard skin on the soles and toes. They are commonly found on the small toes and are caused by pressure points when wearing tight shoes. Use well broken-in shoes for training and apply corn pads to help relieve the pressure. If you have a serious problem with corns, see a chiropodist.

Sprains

Sprains happen when a joint is pushed beyond its normal limitations of movement. The ligaments supporting the joint become overstretched and some of the fibres may even tear. However, they do not break completely and the structure of the joint remains, for the most part, intact. Sprains are extremely painful and will cause swelling and sometimes even a haematoma around the area affected. The joint becomes severely weakened, losing its ability to support weight, and sometimes even its ability to move. Because of these symptoms, severe sprains are often confused with having broken a bone. In cases like these, the only way to be sure is to get to a hospital and have an X-ray. Very severe sprains or injuries in which the ligaments have been completely torn will require hospital treatment, which usually involves the injured part being operated on, splinted or put in a cast.

Less severe sprains should immediately be treated by rest, ice, compression and elevation. You should rest the injured part in an elevated position and apply a cold compress – a bag of frozen peas, for example, wrapped in a towel is ideal. Then tape the injury, but not too tightly, to inhibit further swelling. Once the swelling has decreased, usually about after 24 hours, heat can then be applied to relieve any pain and to help the circulation.

Cramp

Cramp is an extremely painful but luckily not a particularly serious condition which doesn't usually last for very long. It occurs when a muscle (or muscles) suddenly goes into an involuntary contraction, becoming hard and rigid. Cramps can affect any muscle but most commonly occur in the calf muscles and seem to happen either when at rest after strenuous exercise, or at night. Any activity that makes you sweat, or any activity undertaken in hot weather will increase your chance of getting a cramp due to the loss of salt and water in the body. Usually the pain disappears within a few minutes and until then a certain amount of relief can be gained by gently massaging the area.

Chafing

Chafing is caused by friction against the skin. This can be due either to material or else contact with another

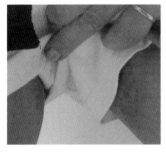

area of skin. It is usually experienced either in the armpits, the groin or on the nipples, and in the worst cases can be very painful. The material of a vest or T-shirt rubbing constantly against the sensitive area can cause chafing of the nipple. To stop it, change your vest or T-shirt to one with softer material and use Vaseline as a lubricant. If you are a long way from home and it is becoming unbearable, rip a small hole out of the material in the nipple area.

Chafing of the armpits or the groin is usually caused by the rubbing of skin against skin, especially during a repeated movement, although clothing can also cause friction here too. As before, the remedy is a good application of petroleum jelly, but make sure that you apply it before you exercise. If you let the chafing continue without treatment, not only will it become very sore, but it may also become infected, which would disrupt your exercise programme.

Rucksack Abrasion

Rucksacks can produce sore spots or abrasions on the back and shoulders if they are badly fitted, badly packed, too heavy or poorly padded. The common areas where abrasions occur are the shoulders, waist (around the kidney area) and the lower back. First of all, always choose a rucksack that fits your body properly; that way you should be able to shoulder the pack for the whole of your route without really feeling it. If at any point you feel any abrasions beginning to develop, try and adjust the straps so that the pack sits better on your back and shoulders. If this doesn't help, identify where the abrasions are at their worst and add extra padding of some kind. Use petroleum jelly to ease the friction and soothe any soreness.

NATURAL HAZARDS

Many people underestimate the dangers present in nature. Any trek off the beaten track will need thorough preparation so that you will know what to do if you get into any difficulties. The first thing to be aware of is the weather: it can change without warning from a beautiful sunny day to cold rain, snow or fog. Fog, in particular, can leave you lost and disorientated. Secondly, terrain can cause problems: rocky ground or rivers can be dangerous, and a walk in the mountains may prove to be more arduous than first thought. Injuries, or even illness, can occur without warning and you may be in a remote place where you will be unable to summon help.

SEVERE INJURY

Although hillwalking is relatively safe it is possible that someone in your party may suffer a serious injury or become ill, for example, a heart attack. The casualty must be thoroughly checked for any injuries or conditions that may be life-threatening, high blood-loss or acute respiratory failure. Assess if there are further dangers (rock-fall) in the immediate area, either to the casualty, yourself or other members of the party. If so, are you able to move the patient without further injury? At all costs avoid unnecessary treatments or moving the patient when there is any danger of spinal injury, as this could have disastrous consequences. It is important to keep the patient as comfortable and as warm as possible, so if shelter and a source of warmth are available, make use of them, ensuring that the casualty is well insulated.

Make arrangements for the prompt removal of the casualty to hospital. If the injury is extremely serious, such as a spinal injury, specialized medical assistance will be required before the casualty can be moved. In these cases, outside help in the form of a mountain rescue team will be needed.

TRAINING AT ALTITUDE

At elevations below 5,000 feet there is hardly any effect on a healthy person, however for those who wish to climb higher there is the added risk of a reduced oxygen supply. The effect is increased with additional height gained and is more noticeable in those people who are unfit or those over the age of 40. Most people can become acclimatized to heights up to 7,000 feet, this is simple a matter of remaining at high altitude. The recommended time is around 3 to 4 weeks during which time you should carry out a normal fitness programme with the emphasis mainly on aerobic exercise. Before acclimatization is complete, some people at high altitudes may suffer acute mountain sickness. This includes such symptoms as headache, rapid pulse, nausea, loss of appetite, and an inability to sleep.

High Altitude Sickness

Altitude sickness (also known as acute mountain sickness) can affect anyone who walks, skis or climbs in high mountains. Although the proportion of oxygen (21 per cent) in the atmosphere remains the same at all altitudes, the air becomes much thinner the higher you go resulting in less oxygen. At 5,000 feet (1,500 m) the oxygen is 80 per cent of its value at sea level. While this might not seem significant it starts to starve the muscles of oxygen and any physical demands on the body become difficult. Humans have difficulty operating in oxygen levels of 70 per cent of norm, because the breathing rate has to be increased to compensate, which in turn reduces the amount of carbon dioxide removed from the blood.

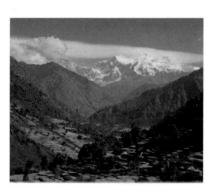

High-altitude sickness is a real danger over 8,000 feet

The symptoms can appear within a few hours when at a height of around 7,000 feet (2,100 m) or more. The higher and quicker you go the greater the symptoms, and the age of the individual also makes a difference. Symptoms include nausea, headache, vomiting and rapid heartbeat, and breathing becomes increasingly difficult.

The sickness becomes dangerous if allowed to persist,

leading to an increased intensity of the symptoms and the additional loss of balance and difficulty in walking. Above 8,000 feet (2,500 m) the lungs can become filled with a frothy fluid – pulmonary edema – resulting in compromised air exchange and shortness of breath.

Altitude sickness can be prevented by acclimatization prior to your excursion, but this can take several weeks. Where acclimatization has not taken place, slowing the rate of ascent will help the body adjust. For those that wish to climb above 8,000 feet (2,500 m) a drug call Diamox will help prevent high mountain sickness. However, taking Diamox can cause symptoms which are similar to those of altitude sickness. Oxygen may be given as an emergency treat-ment but the only real cure is a slow descent to a safe altitude.

AIR POLLUTION

In many cites and towns the air is heavily polluted, particularly with carbon dioxide, carbon monoxide, sulphur oxides and hydrocarbons. When carbon monoxide is inhaled it affects the human body by binding to the hemoglobin in the red blood cells and reducing the amount of oxygen that can carried. Likewise sulphur oxide can irritate the air passageways in the lungs, causing breathing problems.

There is no real answer to combat air pollution while exercising in particularly bad areas. However, try to avoid running in the street during rush hours and exercise in the early morning when pollution is at its

lowest. On days when the contamination is
exceptionally heavy you are advised to stick to indoor
exercise or travel away from the city.

TRAINING ALONE

To be safe, never go it alone in any isolated area, no
matter how much you love the solitude. A walking
partner could prove invaluable in times of difficulty,
especially if you sustain a life-threatening injury or
become unconscious. Make sure that you are properly
dressed and equipped. Make sure that your footwear
is up to the job and that your rucksack carries
camping equipment. Make sure, also, that you are
physically able to do the trip. A good knowledge of
first aid could prove invaluable in an emergency.
Despite the above advice there will still be people who
will insist on walking alone. If you are one of these, it
is essential to follow a few simple rules:

➤ Always leave a copy of your route and and
  estimated time you can be expected back. Leave
  this with someone you know to be responsible.

➤ Consider taking your mobile phone along.
  Although they don't work in many remote areas,
  some mountainous places will have radio relays
  on top of them. Make sure you have the numbers
  of the rescue services programmed into the
  phone or taped onto the back. In an accident,
  this could save your life.

DEHYDRATION

Water makes up the largest proportion of our bodies

– around 75 per cent. It is essential to the proper functioning of the body that it is kept at this level. Problems will start when about two pints are lost and if this isn't replaced the more serious condition of heatstroke will occur, which can lead to death. Dehydration occurs when bodily fluid lost through perspiration, breathing, urination and excretion is not replaced. Therefore it is essential to drink when undertaking any form of exercise that causes excessive sweating, or if the weather is hot.

To reduce the risk of fluid loss, especially if you do not have access to plentiful supplies of good drinking water, you will need to conserve the water already in your body. Make sure that you cover up any exposed skin: not only will this help retain water, it will also protect you against sunburn. Rest as much as possible in the hottest part of the day and limit any activity. Try and find shelter, or attempt to build yourself a basic one. Finally, avoid smoking or drinking alcohol as this will only serve to dehydrate you further.

HEAT EXHAUSTION

Heat exhaustion or heatstroke is a potentially serious condition caused when the body overheats. This can easily happen if you are exerting yourself in hot, dry conditions. The symptoms are weakness and dizziness, the skin may be cold and clammy to touch. Immediate treatment is to get into some shade and rest. The body needs to be cooled as quickly as possible. Make sure clothing is loosened so that air can circulate and pour some cold water over the head and neck. Any lost fluid must be replaced by drinks of

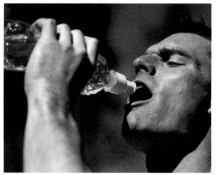

water, if possible with a little salt added. Rest is recommended until recovery takes place, but then things must be taken very slowly or else it could happen again.

SALT DEPLETION

An average human body needs 10 gms of salt a day to help it function; if the levels fall below this, problems will result. Salt is next in importance to water as it helps to control the homeostasis of the body. Sweating can cause a depletion of salt in the body as sweat contains salt as well as water. Salt deficiency is characterized by muscle cramps, nausea, weakness and a hot, dry sensation in the body. As with heatstroke, at the first sign of salt depletion rest in the shade and drink a mug of water, to which has been added a small pinch of salt. If you feel salt loss and dehydration might be a problem on your trip, carry a couple of sachets of rehydration powder in your first-aid kit.

COLD

Exposure to the cold can be deadly. Temperatures below freezing combined with wet and wind create the perfect conditions for hypothermia or frostbite to strike. Wind, in particular, has a severe effect on temperature because the cooling effects of cold air are increased by its movement. This is known as wind chill. For example, air moving at 30 mph (48 km/h) and having a temperature of -20°C (-4°F) has the same chilling effect as air at -40°C (-104°F) moving at only 5 mph (8 km/h). If the weather is wet as well, this will make matters worse as water will help to remove heat from the body. Wet

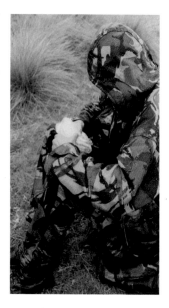

clothes lose their insulating properties.

To combat the threat of hypothermia, use the layer system of clothing as detailed on page xxx, as this will help to trap more warm air close to your body and can also be adjusted to avoid sweating. Sweating needs to be avoided because, like rain, it will reduce the insulation levels of your clothes and conduct your body heat away to the outside. It will also cool the skin. Remember: do everything you can to keep dry, and if your clothes do get wet, either dry them, or get into some dry ones as soon as possible.

Hands and feet, in particular, need to be looked after in the cold. They are the parts that receive the circulation last and are therefore the first to lose it when they get too cold. Make sure that you do not restrict the bloodflow to them by having fastenings at the wrists and ankles too tight, and keep them dry as much as you can. Be aware of any signs of numbness and keep the parts moving. If you need to warm your hands, do so under your armpits or between your thighs. Feet can be kept warm by wriggling the toes, although if they have slight frostbite they can be warmed against a companion. If there are no serious signs, give them a gentle massage. Do not, however, expose any frost-nipped parts to direct heat.

Always carry a spare pair of socks to change into in case yours become wet. In any case, a change of socks once a day will keep your feet in good, hygienic condition. Every now and again, take your boots and socks off and give your feet a massage for about ten minutes. Plastic bags placed over walking boots will add extra insulation, but be careful not to slip.

Hypothermia

Once body temperature falls below 35°C (95°F), the body starts to suffer from hypothermia. With body heat being lost faster than it can be replaced, the organs of the body begin to slow down until, if nothing is done, death occurs. You are at most danger of hypothermia when you are cold, wet, tired, injured or ill. Conditions such as inadequate clothing, immersion in cold water and a lack of food or drink will all exacerbate this condition. The symptoms come on very gradually, so it is not always easily diagnosed. However, you will need to be aware if you, or anyone else, are subject to the conditions

HYPOTHERMIA SYMPTOMS

➤ Uncontrollable shivering

➤ Pale, dry skin which is sub-normally cold to the touch

➤ Muscular weakness and tiredness

➤ Apathy

➤ Irrational behaviour

➤ Change in personality; for example, a quiet person may become aggressive

➤ Eyesight failing

➤ The need to sleep

➤ Slow, weak pulse

➤ Slow, shallow breathing

➤ Eventual collapse and unconsciousness; possible cardiac arrest

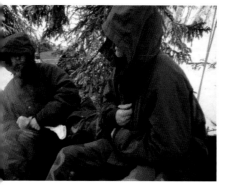

At the first suspicion of hypothermia, everything possible must be done to restore the lost body heat. The casualty needs to rest, out of the cold and wet. Get into some type of shelter if possible, or construct a simple one out of whatever materials are to hand. Wet clothes need to be replaced with dry ones as soon as possible as they will reduce the body heat further. This is particularly important if the casualty has been submerged in water. All clothing in this case will need to be removed as these will kill the sufferer quicker than by just being naked.

The casualty can be warmed in a variety of ways. If she is conscious, and you have the means, get her to eat or drink something hot. Those who constantly exercise outdoors should carry a metallized survival blanket, which is wonderful for warming a hypothermia victim. These blankets are certainly worth considering as they hardly take up any room in your rucksack and yet can be lifesavers. If another healthy person is present, they will also be able to help warm the casualty by sharing their own body heat.

When hypothermia reaches a certain stage, the casualty may become unconscious. If there are no signs of breathing or a pulse, start resuscitation techniques immediately, but don't neglect to keep the sufferer warm. Resuscitation should still be undertaken even if the body temperature has fallen below 26°C (78.8°F), which is when death usually occurs. Even at this stage you cannot assume they are dead and give up. Use assisted ventilation and chest compressions until the body's temperature gets back to normal. If you still cannot revive her after that then she is most likely dead.

Any casualty suffering from either hypothermia or frostbite will need to be handled very carefully, because frozen skin and flesh are extremely delicate and prone to damage. There are several things you can do that will help, as well as certain things that will cause further damage:

HYPOTHERMIA SYMPTOMS

➤ Provide shelter from the wind and cold as soon as possible.

➤ Do not rub or massage to stimulate circulation.

➤ Do not warm the casualty by using external fire or heat.

➤ Give hot food or drink if the casualty is conscious. Chocolate and other high-calorie foods are also good.

➤ Do not allow the casualty to drink alcohol.

➤ The casualty must not exert himself in anyway.

➤ If dry clothing or covering is available, use it to replace any wet clothing.

If it is necessary to replace wet clothing, it should be done piece by piece so that only one part of the body is uncovered at any one time. If you do not have any spare dry clothing, but do have a sleeping or a survival bag, leave the casualty in his or her wet clothes and place them in the bag. Make sure that it is both windproof and waterproof and that it will retain or reflect body heat. This will ensure that the casualty will not lose any more heat, and, at the very least, will stay stable. If another healthy person is available, they can help by sharing the same survival bag and giving some of their body heat to the casualty.

Calorie-counted Menus and Foods

For most people eating is one of the most pleasurable facets of human life. However, when we are dieting or participating in excessive exercise our food demands differ. If we are dieting then our goal is to reduce body fat. We have seen in the previous chapters that restricting calorie intake while increasing exercise activity does this. At the other end of the scale participating in excessive exercise demands a higher calorie intake to maintain the body's nutritional balance. Although we deal with both situations separately, there are only two rules that should always be adhered to: always eat a wide range of foods; and keep to your daily calorie allowance. By doing so you will ensure an adequate intake of all the body's nutritional requirements.

DIET CONTROL

If we are honest with ourselves, no-one really enjoys dieting, nevertheless for some of us it is a necessity. Yet there is no reason why the limited food we consume should be boring. All food should be pleasurable to the palate and well presented. Avoid an all fruit and vegetable diet because of the high water

content which eventually can lead to malnutrition.
Additionally, the body will need some fat.

It is not within the scope of this book to detail a
whole host of menus, but to get you started I have
outlined some sample menus which are listed below.
As we all enjoy different tastes it is up to the you what
you actually consume and the range of low-calorie
meals is only limited by your imagination. When you
eat take time to savour the taste and try to avoid
rushed meals. A few simple tips will help reduce the
calorie intake and still provide an appetizing meal:

REDUCING CALORIES

➤ Reduce portions or bulk out with low-calorie
foods.

➤ Drink water or low-calorie drinks.

➤ Avoid sugar-rich sauces, use reduced fat
dressings.

➤ Use skimmed milk.

➤ Boil or poach foods, rather than grill or fry.

➤ Substitute sugar with sweeteners.

➤ Reduce salt intake.

➤ Avoid alcohol with meals.

Your diet can be helped by restricting the calorie
count according to meal type. For example, breakfast
300, lunch 300, dinner 600, drinks 300; total intake
1500 calories. An example of this would be:

➤ Breakfast: fresh orange juice, poached egg on wholemeal toast.

➤ Lunch: tuna sandwich, bottle of spring water and apple.

➤ Dinner: Fitness Stew (see p.237), low-calorie flan, glass of spring water.

➤ Drinks: $1^{1}/_{2}$ Pints of beer or 2 small tots of spirits

PREPARE YOUR OWN FOOD

The reason for preparing your own food is firstly you control the amount and secondly you control the preparation and the ingredients. The volume of food we eat will depend on what weight loss we are trying to achieve and the type of food being prepared. In using food volume to control weight loss one must be careful that you do not under-eat and deprive your body of vital nutrients and vitamins. The type of food being prepared is also important, meats are generally high in protein where vegetables are not. We must also take into consideration

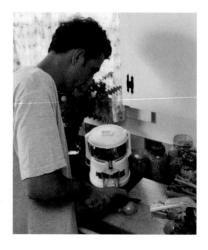

ingredients such as cooking oils, dressing, sources, salt and other additives. Wherever possible use fresh produce. Choose lean meat and healthy looking vegetables and fruit; if fresh is not available use frozen. Avoid eating prepacked, preprepared or tinned meals when on a diet as they contain too many preservatives.

BULKING MEALS WITH VEGETABLES

Although supplying the required calorific value, many diets lack substance, especially when it comes to appearances and size. The restaurant trade found the ideal solution to this many years ago – add lots of colourful salad. Not only does this brighten the appearance but is also bulks out the meal while adding minimal food value.

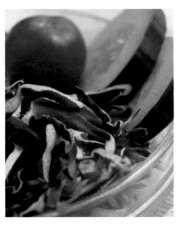

Eating salad as a main meal is also a good idea, though the appearance somehow lacks body. One way around this problem is to convert you plain salad into a sort of ploughman's lunch or a Greek mese. Its easy to get carried away with the amount of relish, cheese, taramasalata and humus so try to keep these to a minimum and improve the salad by adding pickled onions, beetroot and tuna fish.

FRUIT

The benefits of eating one or two portions of fruit
each day are enormous. Fruit contains hardly any
saturated fats and is rich in fibre. Added to breakfast
cereals it helps take away the taste of eating all those
dry and unpalatable bran flakes, and it makes a great
snack if you are feeling hungry or just peckish
between meals.

Best Meal: mixed fruit salad is an excellent meal,
either for breakfast or as a dessert after your main
meal (a $10^1/_2$ oz – 300g – portion is around 150
calories).

BREAD

Despite what other diet books say, and provided you
stay within the recommended daily intake (3 slices
while dieting, 6 slices normal), bread is a versatile
food platform. Almost everyone over the age of two
eats some bread every day, either with a meal
(bulking) or as a sandwich snack. It can accompany
every kind of food – salad, vegetables, meat, cheese,
jam and so on. A large (British) slice of bread is
around 80 calories for wholemeal and 110 for white.
The following sandwiches are a guide based on two
slices of wholemeal bread spread lightly with
polyunsaturated margarine. If you want to liven up
your sandwich use pickles, which average around 130
calories per $3^1/_2$ oz (100 g) opposed to mayonnaise
which contains some 700 plus calories.

SAMPLE SANDWICHES

Sample Sandwiches

Beetroot sandwich = 258 calories
Boiled egg sandwich = 377 calories
Cottage Cheese and tomato sandwich = 290 calories
Ham sandwich = 320 calories
Strawberry jam sandwich = 350 calories
Bacon sandwich = 690 calories
Corned beef sandwich = 437 calories
Chicken sandwich = 348 calories
Tuna sandwich = 290 calories

EGGS

While eggs are full of saturated fats, they are also full
of goodness. A single boiled/poached egg is around
120 calories and with a slice of toast it makes a tasty
and filling breakfast. It is best to restrict your egg
intake to a maximum of four eggs per week, while
taking part in any dietary programme, and six per
week under normal conditions.

Best Meal: pick a small bowl of fresh nettle leaves and
boil for about 20 minutes (substitute spinach if you
can't find any nettles). Remove all the liquid by
pressing with a clean cloth and fry for five minutes in
a little olive oil, then scramble in one or two eggs
during the last minute. Season to taste and serve on

toast. It's tasty, full of protein, iron and fibre, very filling and totals only 350 calories.

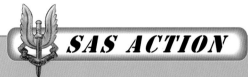

SAS ACTION

➤ During my days in the SAS we were sent to the far-flung corners of the world, living for the most part on 'Compo' – tinned rations to the non-military mind. There was no bread with which to eat the canned jam or cheese – so I made my own using an ammunition tin on top of two Primus stoves for an oven. The yeast we had sent in, the flour I begged from the local Arabs, and the rest of the ingredients could be found in the military 'Compo' pack.

MEATS

For years the SAS have maintained a secret love affair with curry. This came about during the long treks into the dark jungles of Borneo where the only food they had was what they carried. For the most part military rations those days consisted primarily of dehydrated and totally tasteless meat. So the odd natural sweet potato, bamboo core, onion or pepper was added along with several spoonful of curry powder. Although military rations have advanced to the point where

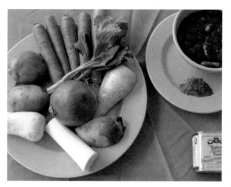

dehydrated food has been replaced with highly advanced freeze-dried products, the SAS curry culture still remains. As an aid to healthy living, curry can convert vegetables into a tasty and nourishing main meal. This conversion, due to its colour and opacity, helps mask the fact that there is little or no meat in the dish.

Best Meal: 7 oz (200 g) of lean beef, chicken and/or mixed hard vegetables (potatoes, carrots etc.) cut into cubes.

1 chopped onion
1 stock cube
3 large tablespoons of curry powder
$2^1/_2$ pints (1.5 litres) of water

Slightly brown the chopped onion in a little olive oil and add the meat and curry powder stirring for about two minutes. Pour into a large saucepan, pour in the water and mix in the stock cube, and bring to the boil. If you wish to add vegetables to bulk it out, add them now and simmer for about two hours, stirring occasionally. Leave overnight so that the curry spices have time to mellow and serve with plain rice. Depending on if you added vegetables or not, this meal will supply four ample servings, which you can either share or freeze for later use. Energy value per serving, including rice, is between 365 and 400 calories.

FITNESS STEW

The one major problem with dieting is the feeling that the food we consume lacks real body – but not with my fitness stew. It looks like a real meal, tastes like a real meal and is highly nutritious. More importantly it will satisfy your hunger and you will have the satisfaction of consuming only fresh ingredients. Try to limit the amount of starchy vegetables you use because the better the mix, the better the taste. Prepare as below – its delicious.

FITNESS STEW

one pack of mixed vegetables, or select your own.

$10^1/_2$ (300 g) of lean meat, pork, beef or lamb (not chicken)
2 Oxo cubes.
$2^1/_2$ pints (1.5 litres) of water.

Chop the vegetables and meat into mouth-sized pieces and add to the water. Crumble the Oxo cubes and bring the whole lot to the boil for five minutes then simmer on a low heat for about two hours. Do not thicken or use extra salt. The meal will provide three large servings, which you can either share or freeze. Energy value per serving is 380 calories.

OUTDOOR EATING

The latter part of this book demands that much of the exercise is conducted outdoors over hilly terrain, where your body will require nourishment to meet the extra energy demand. Fresh food for consumption while walking your routes can consist of sandwiches, fruit or a preprepared meat held in a sealed picnic box. Many people also now prefer to carry packs of freeze-dried food (it's what the SAS carry) while walking over the hills. This type of food has improved dramatically over the past few years and is ideal for camping due to its low weight. The packs contain 96 per cent real food, as opposed to 80 per cent water in wet foods. They are normally packed in a foil pouch that enables boiling water to be added, thus reconstituting the contents hot in the bag. The food can also be cooked normally on a heat-source and by adding water.

SUMMARY

Remember regular exercise and a sensible diet is the only way to achieve weight loss. While the initial process may be hard and take quite a long time, the benefits are a healthier and prolonged life. A fitter body also produces a fitter brain, providing clear thought that will help improve your lifestyle. Define your aim, find the determination to achieve it and the confidence to maintain it. Finally, do not let fitness dominate your life. If there is a special occasion, enjoy yourself, because life without happiness is no life at all.